Herbal Horse Care For Homesteaders

Using natural herbs for the prevention and treatment of horse health concerns

DR. AMANDA P. CARTWRIGHT

Acknowledgments

I would like to thank Rick and Jane Austin for giving me a chance. You had faith in me and I will never be able to say thank you enough for the opportunity to be a speaker at Prepper Camp. It is an honor to be your friend. (www.preppercamp.com)

Many thanks to Dr. Patrick Jones. Your knowledge and way of teaching is how I have learned. I have learned more from you in your online herbal school than I ever did in all of my many years of graduate work to become a doctor of natural medicine. (https://bit.ly/3Io3YOd)

I am grateful to Jeremiah, my husband, who thinks I'm crazy (but I'm not the one who married me...) but still does this insane thing called life with me.

I am also appreciative to my sister, Rachel, for how you cope with your chaotic life as a mother, teacher, caretaker, and role model. You are definitely admired. I don't know how you don't break under all the pressure. You're a very strong individual.

And last but not least, to all the current and future world leaders, I hope you know what you are doing. I refuse to allow my freedom to be taken away because you can't stand strong against money, control, and power. Stop lining your pockets to go along with corrupt agendas. Don't be manipulated. Learn from history. Grow some balls.

Disclaimer:

The publisher and the author are providing this book and its contents on an "as is" basis and make no representations or warranties of any kind with respect to this book or its contents. The publisher and the author disclaim all such representations and warranties, including but not limited to warranties of healthcare for a particular purpose. In addition, the publisher and the author assume no responsibility for errors, inaccuracies, omissions, or any other inconsistencies (including endnotes) herein.

The content of this book is for informational purposes only and is not intended to diagnose, treat, cure, or prevent any condition or disease of an animal. You understand that this book is not intended as a substitute for consultation with a licensed veterinarian. Please consult with your own veterinarian regarding the suggestions and recommendations made in this book. The use of this book implies your acceptance of this disclaimer.

The publisher and the author make no guarantees concerning the level of success you may experience by following the advice and strategies contained in this book, and you accept the risk that results will differ for each animal.

CONTENTS

About the Author

I am a Naturopathic physician. I am not a veterinarian. I have spent countless hours in my graduate studies training to treat and diagnose humans, but not animals. My eyes were opened to a different aspect of using herbal remedies with animals when I began taking courses through the Homegrown Herbalist School of Botanical Medicine. As a Naturopathic physician and veterinarian, Dr. Patrick Jones teaches online courses that are easy to understand and extremely helpful. You can take the lifetime access courses at your own pace and he is constantly adding more classes. I must say, I learned more from his school than I ever did in my doctorate of Naturopathic physician training. His herbology knowledge is impeccable and I highly recommend you going through his school. The knowledge you get will be something you can take and use for the rest of your life. That wisdom will not only help you and your family, but your animals as well. Plus, if you have questions, he will answer them on the school forums! I am an affiliate with his school, however even if I was not, I would still be highly recommending his school. Through the affiliate link listed below, you can also purchase premade tinctures and/or dried herbs if you prefer not to grow them yourself. They are very high quality.
https://bit.ly/3Io3YOd

Another way my eyes were opened to using herbal medicine with animals is when my husband and I began a self-sufficient thriving homestead. When the 'plandemic' happened in 2020, my husband and I began understanding that we had to stop relying on other people because it could be taken away with a blink of an eye. We relied too much on the water company and the power company and the grocery store. So, we began learning and understanding how the land and animals can provide everything a person needs. All it takes is hard work and wisdom. I am thankful our eyes were opened to learn self-sufficiency and be able to implement it so we know what to do and expect in a SHTF scenario. In the process, we became homestead consultants which we have grown to love. Animals are a big part of living off the land and knowing how to handle their health issues is just another piece of the puzzle.

I am also an author of several books found in many bookstores in America. They are listed below.

125 Survival Herbs For Beginners: Useful Herbs and Plants in A Survival Situation https://a.co/d/dsvlqdu

Boost Your Lazy Immune System: 6 Steps to Better Health and Wellness https://a.co/d/5lmlsH5

Health Assessment and Exam: For Goats https://a.co/d/0Cs6yiX

Health Assessment and Exam: For Rabbits https://a.co/d/aujzRgz

The Following books are or will be published soon and are or will be available for purchase on Amazon, Books-A-Million, Barnes and Noble, and many other bookstores!

Herbal Cattle Care for Homesteaders

Herbal Cat Care for Homesteaders

Herbal Dog Care for Homesteaders

Herbal Goat Care for Homesteaders

Herbal Rabbit Care for Homesteaders

Herbal Sheep Care for Homesteaders

Herbal Chicken Care for Homesteaders

Herbal Pig Care for Homesteaders

Herbal Duck Care for Homesteaders

Herbal Animal Care for Homesteaders: A collection of all the books above!

I urge you to check out our YouTube channel called Survival Homestead Teaching Farm. Subscribe and let us know if you have video suggestions! We teach you about herbs, things that we have learned on our way to becoming homesteaders, and the knowledge to survive when SHTF happens. https://www.youtube.com/@survivalhomesteadteaching farm

As if a doctor, author, consultant, and content creator wasn't enough, I am also an event speaker. I absolutely love educating others at homesteading festivals and events. I have been a speaker at Prepper Camp 2023 (www.preppercamp.com) in Saluda NC and look forward to speaking for as long as they let me. I also look forward to speaking at other events including

Mountain Readiness in Harmony NC at the beginning of May 2024. (https://www.mountainreadiness.com/?ref=-NINwVjMEQq7Is) (Affiliate link) Other events too!

Enough about me....let's talk about herbs and horses! Some horse information in this book may apply to you...some may not. In the end, please take away knowledge that could be of help to you today, tomorrow, or in the future, whether you have the horse currently or not. You never know in a SHTF situation when you may need to barter your knowledge.

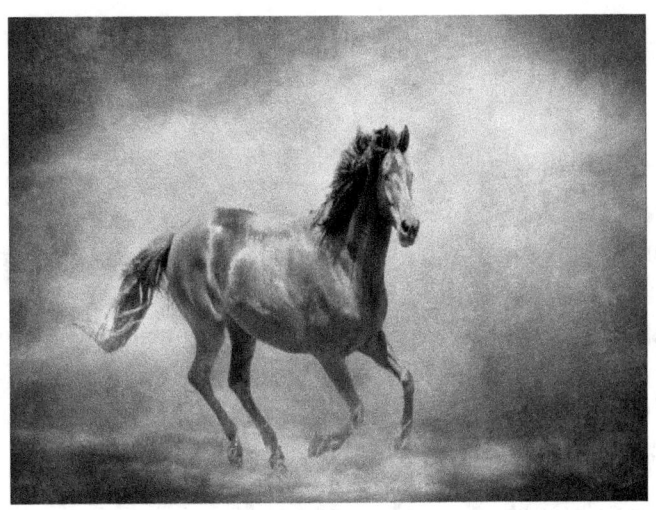

Chapter 1:

Homesteading

Having a homestead to allow complete freedom to live off the land and animals is not easy. A couple hundred years ago, people had to face incredible hardships to build a life. They had no choice because survival was ingrained in them from birth. They grew all their food, had to go to the nearby stream with buckets for all their water consumption and bathing, and figure out how to stay warm through terrible winters. There was a constant threat of disease, fear of being killed by wild animals, and incredible loneliness from being isolated on hundreds of miles of open land (Feek, n.d.).

In modern day, people have become lazy. Most people don't have to work sun up to sun down outside in the scorching sun or in the dead of winter for their families to be fed. Instead, we purchase all our food from grocery stores, rely on the water company to always have water when you turn on the faucet, depend on electricity for heating and cooking, and rest upon knowing a veterinarian will always be a phone call away.

The worry in the past has been about how to stay fed, how to stay warm, and how to stay alive. Today, people have too much ease, too much comfort, and too much spare time. When we want something, we click a button on our phones and it arrives at our doorstep (Feek, n.d.)

Fortunately, with the 'plandemic' (as I like to refer to it), many people are beginning to go back to the old ways where we rely on ourselves instead of others for everything needed for survival. Many are starting to see the grocery store prices surge, they are starting to see how unhealthy processed foods or even store-bought produce really is, and they are starting to follow the money trails and see just how big businesses are not in our best interest.

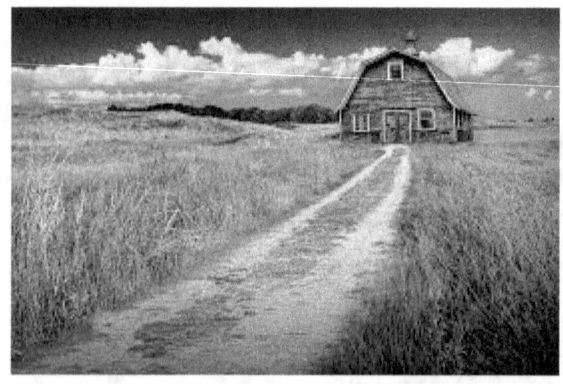

As homesteaders, we want a plot of land, a home of our own, good health, a community we are a part of, hope for our children, and a life filled with meaning and purpose. It's the same as what our ancestors wanted, but we must work hard to beat a system that has trained us to rely on others. We must slow down, reconnect with others, get out of our mind, and find inner peace with being one with our land and animals (Feek, n.d).

My husband and I chose to homestead for many reasons. The uncertainty of how the world is right now is one reason we homestead. We had a growing awareness of storm clouds on the horizon and could see things heading in the wrong direction. We made a choice to avoid catastrophe.

When anyone chooses a homesteading lifestyle, they are going against the mainstream culture. We realized we were in a culture addicted to digital screens, smart devices, and reliant upon others for food and water. We went to the grocery store for food, we drank the water from our tap, never realizing that could all be taken away at some point. That was the catalyst that jumpstarted our homesteading lifestyle. However, we have learned through all the trials and tribulations of the back breaking work, that we are better for it. Better individuals, because its healthy - both physically and mentally. Sunsets mean more, we are thankful for rain, we are grateful for livestock that provide us with so much, and we can truly lift our head and be closer with nature (Feek, n.d.).

Despite what mainstream opinions lead a person to believe, a homestead offers a haven of hope. Believe it or not, your life can improve when you are out of reach of manmade objects and more in tune with nature. Less unhealthy pizza deliveries, less sleepless nights from the sound and lights of cars right outside your windows, and less asphalt and concrete everywhere you look; and more nature experiences such as the serenity of a deer drinking from a pond, a chicken cackling to announce a successful egg lay, or a fragile sprout of a green been pushing out of the soil in a newly planted garden bed (Salatin, n.d.)

On a homestead, you are a part of something bigger; a divine plan of problem solving and perseverance, one in which you are truly free. Free from a world, who many believe is on the verge of destruction (Feek, n.d.).

Having farm animals is a part of homesteading. They can provide a vast array of different types of food including meat, eggs, and milk. On top of that, they provide tender memories that will stay with you for a lifetime. It's a humbling feeling, knowing they rely on you for everything, even love.

When faced with a medical crisis with your animals, you need to understand what to do to help. What medications does the animal need? What dosages? How do I get these medications? Sometimes there just is not time to call a veterinarian. What happens if you do not have the option to call a veterinarian?

Many livestock cannot be taken to your ordinary Veterinarian. Finding a Veterinarian that is knowledgeable in livestock, and willing to come to your homestead can be difficult to find and costly depending upon where you live.

Unfortunately, present day thoughts on medication go straight to pharmaceuticals. People seek out an instant fix with toxic chemicals and vaccines mostly due to lack of time to prepare their own medications for themselves and their animals, the lack of education of alternative remedies, and the power of persuasions of modern commercialism and advertisement. Many have been persuaded to believe artificial remedies is the best route, not realizing the information came from businesses who only have monetary profit in mind.

Cultivating your medications from your own land is not only an amazing, relatively inexpensive, tool for your animals but the fulfillment that you receive by having this knowledge can be accomplishing and satisfying. Being an animal owner means you must have an open mind and be eager to absorb new knowledge and ideas. Herbal comprehension is extensive and will take time to understand, but if you put the work in, it will pay off.

Herbs grow upon the earth for a reason. God put all the medicine on this earth that we as humans or your animals need without having to rely on pharmaceutical medications. Herbs are an important part of nature's chart of wholeness.

Sir Albert Howard, an agriculturist and scientist in the early 20th century, believed that man's neglect of medicinal plants is one of the basic causes of human and animal disease. Herbal medicine can result in remarkable cures.

In fact, pharmaceutical medications are a relatively new thing in the grand scheme of things. Homesteaders/farmers have been relying on herbal cures for thousands of years. We, as a society, have lost that knowledge because we started relying on other people to help instead of helping ourselves.

Animals have been using plants for healing purposes for centuries. It is from observing wild animals that humans learned the healing benefits of plants. For example, in the western United States, Indian tribes learned about the antimicrobial properties of Osha herb by observing bears ingest and roll in the plants. Osha is mainly known and used by humans for its antiviral benefits. It is referred to by many as "bear medicine" (Fisher, n.d.).

There are a number of other interesting discoveries including chimpanzees eating plants to settle their stomachs or chimps using medicinal plants more during the rainy season when they are more susceptible to pneumonia and other diseases. Monkeys even ingest plants to manage fertility including plants that contain isoflavonoids (a compound structurally similar to estrogen) after giving birth to reduce their fertility and when they are ready to give birth, they begin eating a plant called "monkeys ear" that produces a fertility enhancing steroid (Rensberger, 1985).

Have you ever noticed how dogs will know just what type of grass they need to eat when they have an upset stomach. They know how much they need and when to eat it. Their dog parents didn't take them to the side and teach them this knowledge. They just have an ability to know exactly what they need for the problem they are facing.

All animals, including your horse, have an inherent ability to self-select specific plants for use against issues they are facing. They not only know which plant to consume, but they also know how much of that plant to consume to achieve the desired result. This phenomenon is known as Zoopharmacognosy – the study of animals using plants to heal themselves (MacDonald, 2018).

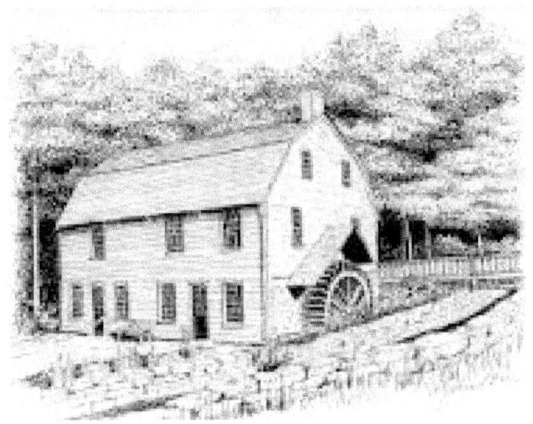

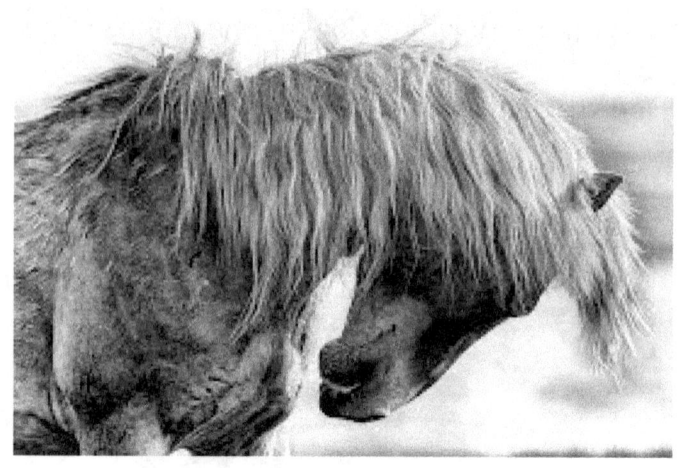

Chapter 2:

Why natural herbs over pharmaceuticals?

God put all the medicine on this earth that we as humans or your animals need without having to rely on pharmaceutical medications. Herbs are an important part of nature and they focus on preventing and treating the root cause of health concerns in humans and horses rather than merely alleviating the symptoms. This approach acknowledges that true healing and long-term well-being can only be achieved when we address the underlying causes of health concerns in your horse.

Unlike the forceful action of pharmaceuticals medications, herbal medication nourishes your horse's specific body system, aiding and assisting his/her body in healing itself. The benefits of herbal medicine are abundant and multifaceted. When you provide your horse with an herbal remedy, your horse often gets healthier due to their nourishing effects. This is not something that can generally be said for using pharmaceuticals with all their harmful side effects.

Synthetic medications are typically expensive and not always readily available. Herbs, on the other hand, are as inexpensive as a pack of seeds, and you can grow as many of them as you like and have room for in your yard.

You can grow your own medicine for your horse. You can't grow pharmaceuticals, although many pharmaceuticals start out as an herbal form. It is then laced with chemicals so big companies can patent it and turn a profit.

Have you ever noticed how one medicine will hurt another function in the body and then you have to take another medicine to counteract the first medicines affects? It is a never-ending cycle. This is what the pharmaceutical companies want. They want you, or your horse, to stay sick. Its more money in their pockets.

In order to understand the effectiveness of herbs, we must delve into the past and understand the history of herbs, veterinarians, and pharmaceuticals. Hundreds of years ago, the homesteader/farmer was an herbalist and a veterinarian all in one. They learned from a young age how to take care of their animals naturally because herbs were the only medicine.

This was knowledge that each person had long before there were doctors who solely took care of animals. None of those animals went extinct. They survived and thrived. So, what changed?

The use of plants as herbs has been important to all cultures since long before history was recorded. Hundreds of tribal cultures have used wild and cultivated herbs for medicinal and food purposes for thousands of years. As civilizations developed, so did the knowledge for the use of herbs as medicine (Coates, 2012).

Physicians in America studied and relied on plants as their primary medicines through the 1930's. Up until the 1930s, medical schools in America taught basic plant taxonomy, pharmacognosy, and medicinal plant therapeutics. Physicians routinely used plant drugs as their primary medicines. In fact, the word "drug" is derived from a word for the root of a plant (PennState Extension, 2023).

A pharmacopoeia is an official publication of medicinal drugs with their effects and directions for usage. In 1870 the United States Pharmacopoeia listed six hundred and thirty-eight herbs in its publication. By 1990 there were only fifty-eight herbs. Now, there are zero herbs listed (USP, 2023).

Some of these plants fell out of use due to their weakness or toxicity. However, the majority of clinically useful plants were replaced by pharmaceuticals which could be patented, thereby capable of generating larger profits as well as supporting conventional medicine (Oakland Veterinary, 2019).

Herbal medicine is a vibrantly alive discipline that is being used actively in many other cultures throughout the world today. There is no question that herbal preparations can be of benefit to you or your horse.

In France and Germany, it has been estimated that thirty to forty percent of all medical doctors/veterinarians rely on herbal preparations as their primary medicines. Unfortunately, the percentages in the United States are close to zero (Woo, 2012).

In the late 1700's veterinarian medicine, as we know it in the modern world, began in Europe. In the mid 1800's, Americans became familiar with veterinarian medicine, however veterinarians were few and far between (Oakland Veterinary, 2019).

Up until 1965, all veterinarians in America used herbs as medicine to treat animals. It wasn't until 1965 that herbal medicine in the veterinarian practice was replaced by pharmaceuticals (Oakland Veterinary, 2019).

From 1965 to present day, pharmaceuticals have been sold to Americans, engraining it into them from birth, that toxic medications are the best and safest way of 'treating' health concerns. While I do agree some pharmaceuticals have their place, most should not be on the market, especially when there are natural herbs that can do the same thing. The food and drug administration states they are safe, however the lasting effects on the body are questionable.

Before the food and drug administration in 1965, veterinarians would fill their yards full of herbs so they would have medicine readily available when they needed (Oakland Veterinary, 2019). There were many benefits to treating animals in a very holistic and natural way. One of which was not having the side effects on the animal's liver as pharmaceuticals typically will enhance.

The liver filters all of the blood in the body and breaks down pharmaceuticals. If your horse is on pharmaceutical medications, how do you know he or she will be able to metabolize those medications adequately? Why not give him/her herbs that you know their liver will be able to handle?

Along with your horse's health, you must look of the bigger picture. Providing pharmaceutical medications to your horse means there are pharmaceutical components in your soil. If you use their manure for compost, then you are putting those pharmaceutical components around your garden and then you are consuming those plants. Do you see the vicious cycle?

Another concern for pharmaceuticals is resistance. Antibiotics especially can become resistant with excessive usage. This means they will not work on your horse when needed. They can, in turn, create gastrointestinal issues, palpitations, and/or seizures, all of which are one-hundred percent unnecessary. Why put your horse though pain when it could be avoided?

There are no doubts veterinarian bills are outrageously expensive. The national average veterinarian bill, consisting of only a house call with general routine maintenance for a horse, is over two thousand dollars a year. That is one big reason to go herbal (Ruff, 2016).

Another reason is the fact that getting a veterinarian to come to your horse stable is a concern for many. You can't just load your horse in your car and haul him to the vet like a dog or cat. Veterinarians who can diagnose and treat large animals are few and far between and they charge an arm and a leg to make house visits if you can find a veterinarian willing to do so.

Those may not be the only reasons you want to treat your horses as naturally as possible. You may choose to go the herbal route for financial reasons. You may choose to go the herbal route for health benefits to your horse. You may choose to go the herbal route because of how the world is changing and becoming so uncertain.

If you are tired of agendas being pushed, especially those in the pharmaceutical realm, consider going back to simpler times, before monetary profit was the biggest goal, and harness the knowledge of herbal medications for your horse.

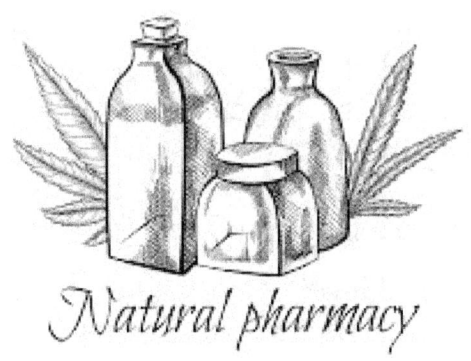

Natural pharmacy

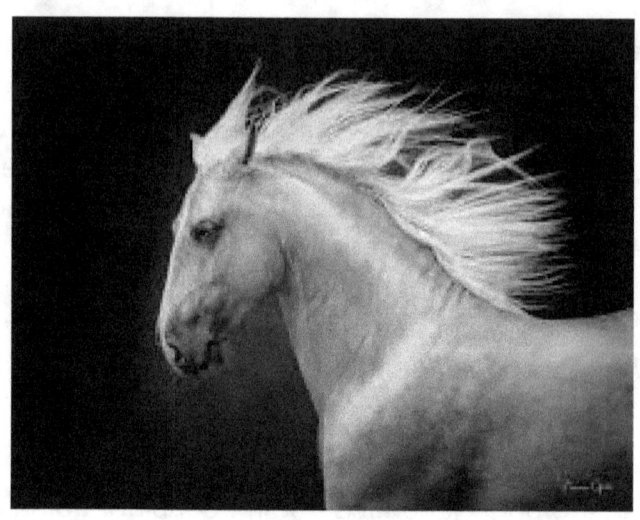

Chapter 3:

Herbal Knowledge

With herbal knowledge, you will be able to treat your horse in times of crisis. If you are able, I would always recommend consulting a veterinarian but with how the world is currently changing, you never know when you will need this wisdom in your back pocket.

In June of 2023, the U.S. Food and Drug Administration mandated all medically important antimicrobials and other general livestock and pet medications to be removed from over-the-counter to prescription only by a qualified veterinarian (U.S. Food and Drug Administration, 2023).

Because of this change, many have been researching and understanding herbal medications better to use on their animals for general use and for crisis situations. While many feel herbal medication is plan 'B', there are many others who have solely used herbal medications on their animals for years and have had great success.

While herbal medications can be used as a preventative or to treat a particular ailment, if your animals are taking any type of pharmaceuticals, you need to air on the side of caution because the herbs and pharmaceutical medication can and will interact with each other. Also, some herbs can be dangerous during pregnancy and lactation.

Herbs have many benefits over pharmaceuticals and are amazing medicine. Pharmaceuticals can be strong and have significant side effects. Using natural medications can reduce your animal's reliance on synthetic toxins and avoid possible side effects. Natural herbal medications are also more accessible. You can purchase dried herbs or grow them yourself. Once you have access to herbs, all you need is the knowledge of how and when to use them.

Wouldn't it be nice to be able to see a problem with your horse, go to your yard and grab a twig of this of sprig of that, and treat your horses without the costly veterinarian bills?

If you purchase dried herbs, you can expect a shelf life of around a year, more if you purchase from a reputable place such as from the Homegrown Herbal School of Botanical Medicine. https://bit.ly/3lo3YOd If you grow and dry an herb yourself, you can expect around a two-year shelf life but the way you dry the herb and store the herb does play a big role in that shelf life.

Ways to dry herbs include using a dehydrator, using a freeze drier, using screens, etc. to air dry over several days. Whichever way you choose, make sure to keep the herbs away from direct sunlight and never dry it above one hundred- and ten-degrees Fahrenheit. This changes the chemical bonds and 'cooks' the herb, making the medicinal benefits disappear. Always wait to grind the herb into a powder until you are ready to use it. This helps keep the medicinal properties intact and prolongs the shelf life.

Depending on the horse, some herbs may be best used fresh. Some herbs are meant to be used short term and some herbs are meant to be used for a longer term. If your horse has a chronic problem and they are consuming an herb long term, it is best to give their body a rest. Every couple of weeks, take a day off and do not give the herb to your horse. This will allow their body to reset. Usually when they resume consuming the herb, the herb works even better at combating the particular ailment.

How much of an herb to give depends on your horse and their needs. It also depends on many other factors such as gender, weight, age, the actual herb, and other foods/medications he or she is already consuming. The treatment dosing listed in this book, except for foul's, is based upon an 1100-pound healthy adult horse.

In many cases, using herbal remedies as a preventative can be of great use to horses. If using as a preventative, take the dosage given as a treatment and divide it in half. Simply give half of what is described to help prevent the health concern from developing.

Some animals are harder than others to get to consume herbal medicine. For livestock, fresh herbs are usually eaten without a second thought and dried powdered herbs mixed into their feed works most of the time. But what about finnicky horses? Sometimes you have to be creative when it comes to giving your horse herbal medicine by mixing it in with their normal feed, making a tea and adding that to their water bucket, making a tincture and adding a few drops to their feed or water, making an herbal oil or salve and rubbing that into a wound or stiff joint, or simply hiding the herb in something delicious they enjoy eating. We will discuss more about teas, tinctures, herbal oils, poultices, and salves in chapter 5.

I must not fail to mention that consuming herbs is not the only route of administration. Topical use can also be applied when the situation allows.

If you decide to grow herbs yourself, there are a great deal of the herbs mentioned in this book can be grown in your yard alongside your decorative flowers. Many of them are perennial so once you plant them, you don't have to worry about saving the seeds and replanting them year after year. Your yard can be full of medicine, but look like a regular flower garden to most.

Planting herbs for your animals can also create a bonus that will allure pollinating bees towards your property and potentially your gardens. The herbs look nice but have functionality too!

Safety

There have been some controversial rumors about the effectiveness and safety of herbs. Obviously, if your horse is pregnant or taking other pharmaceutical medication, be cautious with giving herbs internally.

Comfrey is one herb that has gotten a bad rap in the past few decades. It works really well, however there are many research studies that show how ineffective it may be to your horse. You must take a look at the type of study and how the study was administered to understand herbs, specifically comfrey (Homegrown Herbalist, n.d.)

In one study, six-week-old rats were fed comfrey as forty percent of their diet and some of those rats developed liver tumors (Homegrown Herbalist, n.d.). If you ate only one particular food as forty percent of your diet, without getting other needed vitamins, minerals, and nutrients, you would have problems too!

What the studies failed to do is let us know other factors that could have contributed to the liver tumors. What pharmaceuticals were the rats on at the time of the study? What did the rats diet consist of? Were they ingesting other food additives? How healthy were the rats' livers prior to the study? We don't know because the study didn't take all the factors into consideration. Scientists can say 'research says....' and most of the time people fall for it.

I think it is safe to say that horses should not consume comfrey as forty percent of our diet. I also think it would be wise to not give comfrey to your horse internally at excessively high doses (more than forty leaves per day) or for prolonged periods of time. I would not think negatively about comfrey based on research studies that are not taking all factors into account. Look at the many positive comfrey testimonials of horse owners and draw your own conclusion.

Comfrey isn't the only controversial herb. Many websites claim herbs are unsafe because research on that particular herb is lacking. To be very honest, there are hundreds of years of research with these herbs. Just look at history! Herbs were the medicine of our ancestors and the medicine they gave their livestock to keep them healthy. Maybe looking back on history will help some understand the safety and effectiveness of herbs for their horse.

Many scientific sources claim herbs are bad, only to find out in the end that some scientists are paid to say this in order to push pharmaceutical medications which puts money into certain people's pockets.

It is true that some herbs can cause allergic reactions. The pharmaceuticals do too! With giving herbs to your horse, you need to have a bit of education to know how the herb will affect your horse, proper dosage, and how to prevent the health concern in the first place. This is what this book aims to do!

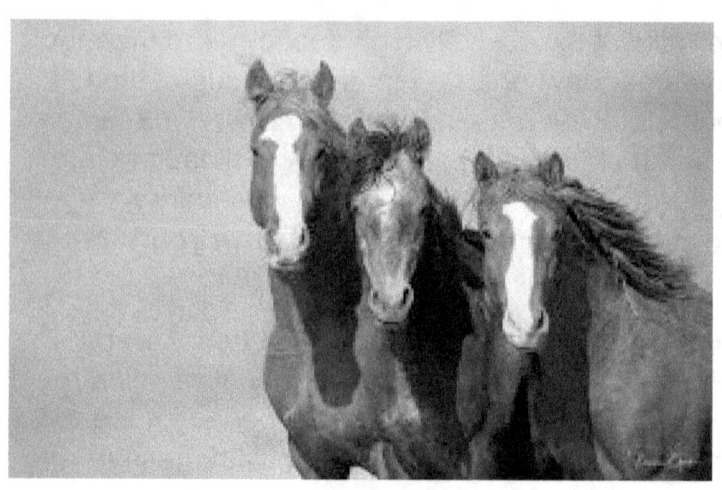

Chapter 4:

How to harvest and dry herbs

Of course, you can purchase herbs. If you do, make sure it is from a reputable place where you know how the herbs have been dried, how long they have been sitting on the shelf, and under what conditions have they been on the shelf. I mentioned the link for the Homegrown Herbalist at the beginning of this book. I do highly recommend them.

If you choose to grow your own herbs, you can have a natural pharmacy just outside your door, many of which will come back year after year. How fantastic would it be to open your door and have your own veterinarian pharmacy at your fingertips? Whether you grow medicinal herbs for horse or you grow herbs as a deterrent for many pests, preventing and treating naturally can potentially save you hundreds of dollars on veterinarian bills and possibly save your horse a lot of hassle with having toxic pharmaceuticals running through their system.

It is best to harvest herbs early in the day, after the dew is gone, but before the hot sun can dry out the oils inside the herb. Only harvest some of the plant to make sure it doesn't die.

If you are harvesting leaves, you will usually cut off small branches, making it easier to dry them. For flowers, wait until they have developed fully and harvest them as soon as possible after they have fully opened. If you are harvesting only the seeds, you will need to wait until the seeds mature and the seed pod dries on the stem before harvesting.

Once you have the herb, you may want to dry the herbs for later use. There are a few ways this can be accomplished. Traditionally, herbs are air-dried without any additional heat source. Heating any herb to one-hundred-and-ten-degrees Fahrenheit or more will kill all the beneficial medicine that lies within the herbs.

Many choose to bundle the herb together by tying the stems with string or a rubber band and hanging them upside-down in a dry place away from light. If you do this, make sure the bundles are in smaller quantity to make sure there is adequate airflow through all the herbs.

Drying racks are another option. This is another way to allow air to dry for three to four weeks without adding heat or allowing light to penetrate the herb. Many will simply lay them on wire racks with a fan on low speed. Others will use old screening material and lay all the herbs out in a single layer so that the herb is getting airflow from all sides.

It is possible to dry herbs with a dehydrator. Ideally the dehydrator should have a fan to circulate the warm air so that the entire batch dries evenly. You must make sure, as stated before, the temperature setting is not at or above one-hundred- and ten-degrees Fahrenheit. This is another reason you must do your due diligence on finding a reputable herb company if purchasing without growing yourself. You need to know how the herb has been dried and how long it has been sitting on the shelf!

You can also dry herbs in a stove, only if you have a proofing oven in which the temperature stays at ninety to ninety-five degrees. Many will say using a sun oven can be used, however I would not recommend this method. While herbs will dry in a sun oven, unfortunately they are subjected to an immense amount of light in the process and that in and of itself can denature the medicinal benefits.

Store your dried herbs in a clean, sealed glass jar away from light. Make sure they are one hundred percent dried before storing. As mentioned before, it is best to wait and crush them into a powder until immediately before using the herb for your horse.

In order to powder the herbs, simply take the herbs and crush with a blender or mash them using a hand-held mortar and pestle. Some may choose to use a spice-mill or coffee bean grinder. Afterwards, you may want to use a fine sieve to make sure everything has been pulverized into a fine powder. This is not one hundred percent needed for your horse, but it may help when making herbs into teas, tinctures, herbal oils, herbal salves, etc.

Even if you don't have the space or simply don't want to grow these herbs, look at the amount of money you would save by purchasing already dried and powdered herbs that ship right to your door versus a veterinarian bill. Of course, if you decide to purchase herbs, you need to make sure they are from a reputable source.

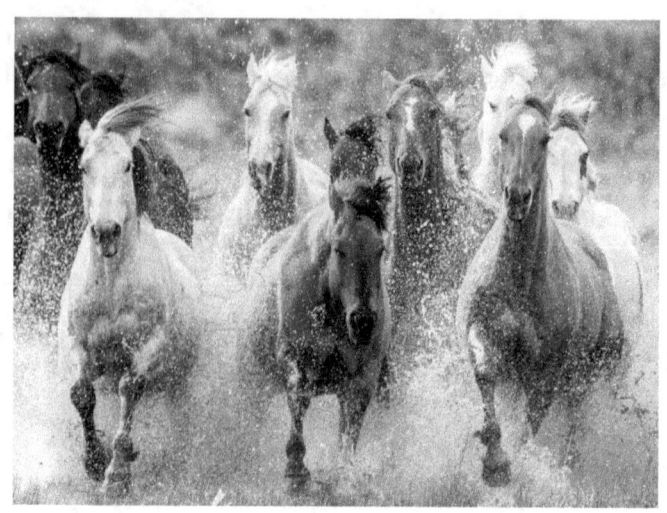

Chapter 5:

How to use herbs medicinally

When it comes to herbal medicine, there is no shortage of options for reaping the bountiful benefits of these natural wonders. From tinctures to salves, a poultice, oils, and teas, each delivery method offers a unique way to harness the healing powers of medicinal herbs that promote overall well-being.

Once you have those herbs dried and powdered, what do you do with them? Sometimes your horse will enjoy the new taste and devour it without giving you grief. Sometimes you might not get so lucky. There are many ways to process herbs. I'll take you through a few steps briefly so you will know exactly what to do.

Herbal infusions/decoctions (Tea)

A tea, also known as an infusion or decoction is taking an herb and infusing it into water. Using an herbs' leaves or flower is called and infusion and using the bark or stems in a more concentrated form of an herb is called a decoction. There are several methods to use and you can infuse more than one herb at a time if desired (Apelian, 2021).

To give an herbal tea to a horse, simply allow it to drink the tea. If the horse seems to not want to drink it, you can always add it to their water bucket in increments. If neither of these options work, you can syringe it into the back of their throat.

Stove method:

1.   To make an infusion, start with cold distilled or purified water in a non-metal cooking pot with a lid. The cold water ensures the maximum amount of beneficial nutrients from the herb(s) are extracted. Use a ratio of four-ounces dried herb(s) to sixty-four ounces water. Let it soak for a few hours in the cold water.

2.   Cover the cooking pot and boil slowly. It must be covered to allow all medicinal benefits to stay inside. Once it begins to boil, decrease the temperature to simmer fifteen to twenty minutes or until the volume of the liquid has reduced to thirty-two ounces.

3.   Strain with a cheesecloth and let it cool. Squeeze herb(s) through the cheesecloth to ensure all liquid has been removed. Pour into a clean glass jar with a lid. This can be stored in the refrigerator for up to two days or it can be frozen.

Cup Method:

1.   Place one ounce of your herb(s) into a sixteen-ounce mug.

2.   Pour boiling water over the top.

3.   Place a lid, plate, or anything you have over the top of the mug. This is very important. This keeps all the medicinal benefits inside the cup and prevents them from escaping.

4.   Allow this to simmer for at least ten minutes but preferably up to two hours.

5.   Remove the lid and strain the herb(s).

6. Use with your horse immediately.

French Press Method:

1.   Place two ounces of your herb(s) into a French press.

2.   Insert the strainer part on your French press with strainer part to the top.

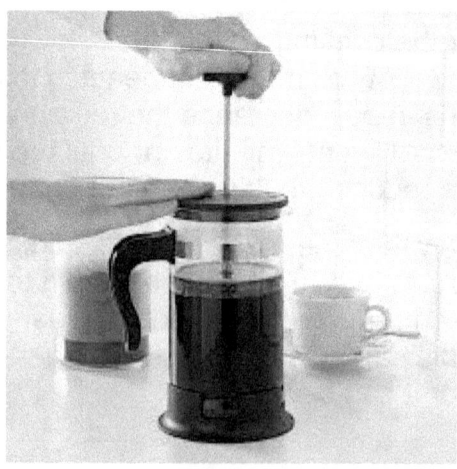

3.   Pour thirty-two ounces boiling water over the top of your herb(s).

4.   Place the lid on the top of the French press but do not push down on the strainer. Leave it up.

5.   Allow this to simmer for at least ten minutes but preferably up to two hours.

6.   After this period of time, push down on the strainer to allow all the herb(s) to be pushed to the bottom of the French press.

7.   Allow the tea to cool before giving to your horse.

Herbal Pills/Balls

Herbal Pills are an easy way to get herbs into a horse. They are dried pill-size balls packed full of herbal goodness (Homegrown Herbalist, n.d.).

Mucilage is a water-soluble edible adhesive material that constitutes carbohydrates and uranic acids units present in different parts of plants including the mucous epidermis of the outer layer of seeds, bark, leaves, and buds. Some herbs high in mucilage include comfrey, marshmallow, and slippery elm (Homegrown Herbalist, n.d.).

1.   Mix nine parts of a dried herb with one part of an herb high in mucilage.

2.   Add a little water to make a stiff dough.

3.   Roll into pill-sized balls.

4.   Dry thoroughly.

5.   Store in a dark place away from heat and moisture.

Herbal Tincture

A tincture is a concentrated liquid herbal extract obtained by steeping dried herbs in alcohol. The alcohol breaks down the plant's cell walls, liberating its bioactive compounds, which are then preserved in the alcohol solution (Apelian, 2021).

To preserve the dried herb(s) indefinitely, the alcohol used should be eighty to one hundred-proof. Vodka is usually the cheapest, has no flavor, and is usually preferred in a tincture, however other alcohols can be used as long as it is at least eighty-proof.

Over the course of four to eight weeks, the dried herb(s) infuses into the alcohol. Some will say differently; however, with a tincture, you always want to use dried herbs, whether they are powdered or not. The moisture content of fresh herbs can damage the longevity of the preservation (Apelian, 2021).

It is worth noting the differences between a tincture and an extract. A tincture uses alcohol whereas an extract uses other liquids such as apple cider vinegar or glycerin. An extract does not have the shelf life of a tincture.

When making tinctures, you can put several herbs into the jar with the eighty to one hundred proof alcohol. However, if you have several different tinctures already made up, you can't add that to the tincture you are making.

To give a tincture internally to a horse, merely place a few drops into their water bucket or use as directed by the particular ailment they are facing. Most people know that tinctures are taken internally but did you know they can be used externally as well?

Topical use of tinctures can help your horse with various wounds, bites, and stings. The amber bottles made for tinctures do sometimes come with spray tops. You put the spray top on the bottle and spray the tincture directly onto the wound, bite, or sting.

One caveat to spraying a tincture is watering it down. Watering the tincture down will help the wound to not burn as much when applying the tincture. If you do water it down, make sure to use good, clean water. I prefer soft rain water. Do not ever use tap water. This is laced with many harmful chemicals. Once you add water to the tincture, it should be used up completely within two days. Add water at a ratio of one part tincture to five parts water.

To give a tincture to a horse, you can add it to their feed or you can add a small amount of clean water and syringe it into the back of their throat.

There are two methods of making tinctures.

Folk Method:

1.   Fill a clean glass jar half full of the dried herb(s) you are using.

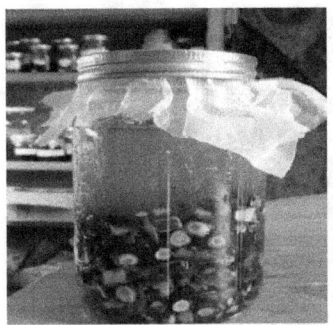

2.   Fill jar with alcohol leaving a half inch headspace in the jar.

3.   Alcohol (or anything acidic) tends to rust metal lids, therefore if you place a piece of

wax paper or parchment paper under the lid before screwing it on, it will keep a barrier there to help avoid rusting.

4.   Once the lid is on, turn it up-side-down to mix well.

5.   Label the jar with the herb(s) used and date the tincture is started.

6.   Keep the jar in a cool, dry, dark location for eight weeks to six months, shaking it daily to mix.

7.   After this time period, strain out the herb through a cheesecloth.

8.   Pour tincture into an amber color bottle. The amber color bottles keep light from entering the bottle. Light will denature a tincture and cause the shelf life to shorten.

Ratio Method: (1 to 5)

1.   Using a scale, set a clean glass jar on top and press 'tare'. This will allow you to measure the exact quantity of herb(s) and alcohol to use.

2.   Use one part herb(s) to five parts alcohol in the glass jar. (This method helps save alcohol) Example: If you use five grams herb(s), use twenty-five grams alcohol.

3.   Alcohol (or anything acidic) tends to rust metal lids, therefore if you place a piece of wax paper or parchment paper under the lid before screwing it on, it will keep a barrier there to help avoid rusting.

4.   Once the lid is on, turn it up-side-down to mix well.

5.   Label the jar with the herb(s) used and date the tincture is started.

6.   Keep the jar in a cool, dry, dark location for eight weeks to six months, shaking it daily to mix.

7.   After this time period, strain out the herb through a cheesecloth.

8.   Pour tincture into an amber color bottle. The amber color bottles keep light from entering the bottle. Light will denature a tincture and cause the shelf life to shorten.

Herbal Oil Infusion

Herbal oil infusions are carrier oils that have had dried herbs soaked in them for a period of time. These are then used topically on your horse. The herbs must be dried because the moisture content of fresh herbs could make the oil go rancid. Herbal infused oils can keep for one to two years if stored properly (Apelian, 2021).

Carrier oils are plant-based oils used to 'carry' the medicinal benefits of an herb onto the horse's skin. These carrier oils that are good for a horse's skin are organic olive oil, sweet almond oil, coconut oil, emu oil, jojoba oil, castor oil, tamanu oil, grapeseed oil, argon oil, apricot oil, avocado oil, lard (from pigs), and tallow (from cattle).

Please do not confuse an herbal infused oil with an essential oil. Essential oils are the oils naturally found in an herb which are extracted. It takes very large amounts of an herb to make a very small amount of essential oil. Essential oils are highly concentrated and so powerful that they should almost never be applied directly to a horse's skin.

Cold Herbal Oil Infusion Method:

1.   In a clean glass jar, fill half way with dried herb(s).

2.   Pour a carrier oil over the herb. Fill within a half inch of the top.

3.   Put lid onto the jar.

4.   Mix well by turning the jar up-side-down.

5.   Label the jar with the herb(s) used, carrier oil used, and the date.

6.   For six to eight weeks, keep the jar in a location away from light and turn it up-side-down at least once a day to mix the herb(s) and carrier oil.

7.   After the six to eight weeks, remove the lid and strain the herb(s) through a cheesecloth. Squeeze the cheesecloth to get all the oil out.

8.   Store in a clean glass jar with a lid in a cool, dry, dark location and label with the herb(s), carrier oil used, and date of completion. You can use immediately on your horse by applying topically to wounds. You can also use this to make an herbal salve.

Hot Herbal Oil Infusion Method: Crockpot

1.   In a clean glass jar, fill half way with dried herb(s).

2.   Pour a carrier oil over the herb. Fill within a half inch of the top.

3.   Put lid onto the jar.

4.   Mix well by turning the jar up-side-down.

5.   Put the jar or jars into a crockpot with a 'warm' setting.

6.   Add about two inches of water to the crockpot. Add more water when necessary to make sure the water level stays consistent throughout the entire process.

7.   Allow the jars to sit in the slightly warm crockpot water for four to seven days.

8.   Remove the jars from the crockpot and allow them to cool.

9.   Strain the herb(s) by using a cheesecloth. Squeeze all the carrier oil out.

10.   Put a lid on and label the jar with the herb(s) used, carrier oil used, and the date of completion. You can use immediately on your horse by applying topically to wounds. You can also use this to make an herbal salve.

Hot Herbal Oil Infusion Method: Double Boiler

1.   Fill a cooking pot half way with water and bring to a boil.

2.   Add your herb(s) and carrier oil to a double boiler and set this on the top of the boiling water. Use a ratio of one part herb(s) to two parts carrier oil.

3.   Turn down the heat of the water and allow the mixture to simmer for four to five hours.

4.   Once the herb(s) have been thoroughly infused into the oil, strain the herb(s) out of the carrier oil

through a cheesecloth. Squeeze the cheesecloth to get all the oil out.

5.   Put a lid on and label the jar with the herb(s) used, carrier oil used, and the date of completion. You can use immediately on your horse by applying topically to wounds. You can also use this to make an herbal salve. While this is a faster method, the crockpot method is still highly recommended.

Herbal Salve:

An herbal salve acts the same as an herbal oil infusion, except it takes on a solid substance that is easier to apply topically to a horse's wounds, skin irritations, or sore muscles. Vitamin E is commonly used in salves to help with rancidity problems; however, it is not a necessary ingredient. You must have an herbal infused oil to make a salve.

Containers that you use for your herbal salve should not be plastic or aluminum. Plastic can melt when you add the salve and it also can seep harmful chemicals into the salve. Aluminum does the same. Aluminum can cause brain, liver, and kidney problems in a horse so it is best to avoid it when possible.

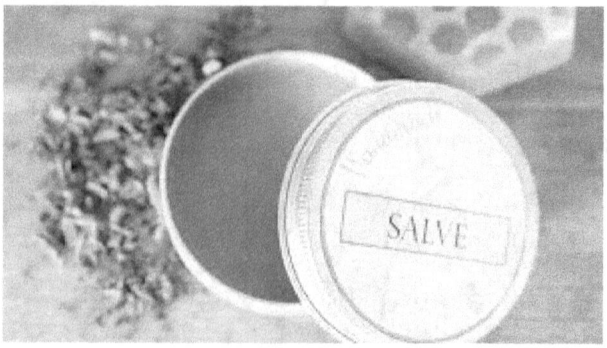

1.   Fill a cooking pot half way with water and bring to a warm simmer (not boiling because you don't want to heat the herbal oil any more than one hundred degrees).

2.   Place one cup of your herbal infused oil into a double boiler on the top of the water.

3.   Add one fourth cup of beeswax.

4.   Add vitamin E oil at this time if desired.

5.   Once the beeswax has melted, mix well and add to your containers.

6.   Allow to cool completely to solidify.

Herbal Poultice:

A poultice can be an effective way of getting a fresh or dried herb to soak into the skin quickly. A poultice is a common topical treatment used on horses, usually used on the lower legs, to help inflammation, wounds, and to pull our toxins from bees, wasps, spiders, or snakes (Apelian, 2021).

A poultice needs to be wrapped to stay in place. A popular type of bandage to keep poultices in place is called Coflex. Coflex is a bandage material that wraps around an area that sticks to itself. Poultices needs to be changed frequently.

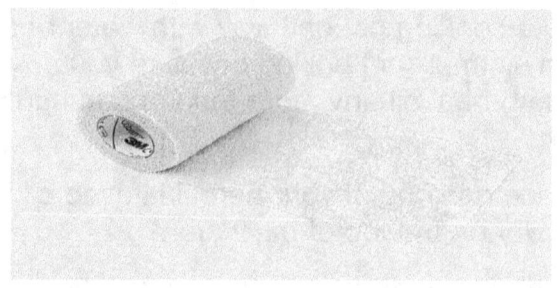

Traditional Method:

1.   Cut or crush the herb(s) up finely. You can do this with a knife, blender, or a mortar and pestle.

2.   Mix with a touch of water to create a mush mixture.

3.   Apply a generous quantity directly onto the horse's skin.

4.   Wrap with a dressing. Change this dressing frequently.

Spit Method:

1.   Put several leaves of the herb(s) you are using in your mouth.

2.   Chew the herbs to a mush and spit out.

3.   Apply a generous quantity directly onto the horse's skin.

4.   Wrap with a dressing. Change this dressing frequently.

Using herbs medicinally is as easy as feeding your horse fresh or dried herbs, making an herbal infusion or decoction tea, preparing an herbal infused oil, making an herbal salve, producing a ready to go tincture, or making an on-demand poultice. Knowing how to use herbs medicinally is a big part of understanding herbal horse care.

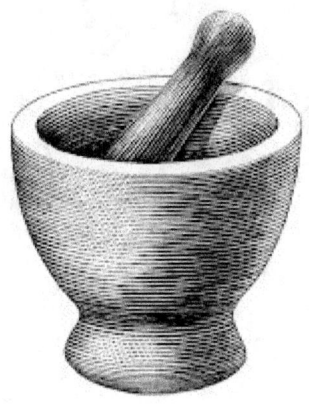

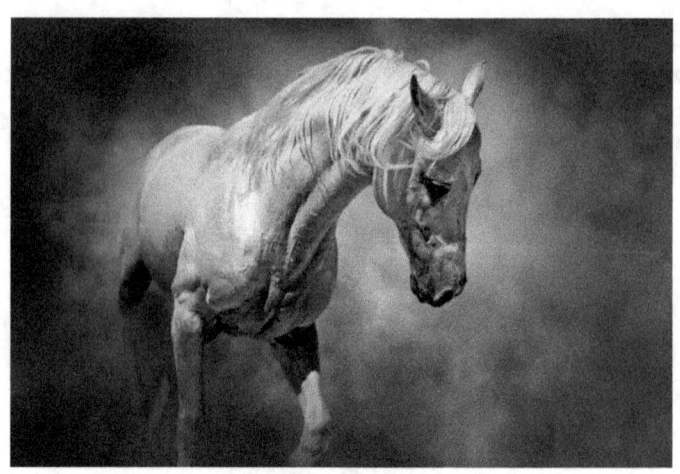

Chapter 6:

Immune System

The immune system is something that needs to be boosted with any type of horse illness. It is so important that it needs its own chapter. The immune system of the horse is a fascinating, complex, and plays a critical role in tackling the infections that it encounters. It is instrumental in protecting the horse when foreign invaders, such as viruses, parasites, fungi, or bacteria, breach the physical barriers—such as skin and mucous membranes—and enter the body (Tizzard, 2022).

Chronic stress, whether physical or mental, weakens the immune system. Age and nutrition are both also closely linked to immunity and immune function. The following vitamins, minerals, and herbs can help boost the horse's immune system.

Vitamin C

A good source of vitamin C is good quality green grass. Commercial grains are not particularly high in vitamin C, but they can have a huge upsurge in Vitamin C if you allow them to sprout. It is suggested that the vitamin C content of oats can be increased by up to six hundred percent when sprouted. Sprouts may be a good way to provide organic vitamin C in times of stress. One herb that is a rockstar for vitamin C that horses may ingest is rosehips (Equinews, 2013).

Vitamin E

Vitamin E is fat-soluble that helps maintain a healthy immune system. Horses need vitamin E because they cannot synthesize it endogenously in their body. Horses that are mostly on lush pasture will get this needed vitamin. Cutting grasses and drying it will cause rapid degradation of vitamin E that continues as the hay is stored (FitAudit, n.d.). If you choose to give a horse a synthetic (not recommended) source of Vitamin E, give a minimum of 4,000 international units per day. Oregano, sage, and cloves are high in vitamin E and are safe for horse consumption (Darani, 2020).

Omega 3 fatty acids

Omega-3 fatty acids are a polyunsaturated fat that a horse cannot produce on their own. Horses must ingest them to receive a balanced diet. Omega-3 fatty acids are found in dark, leafy plants, which are traditionally the cornerstone of the equine diet. Omega-6 fatty acids are also a polyunsaturated fat and are found in the oil of cereal grains and seeds. This means that as horses eat less forage and more grain, they are inherently consuming more omega-6 fatty acids. While horses need both sources of omega fatty acids, a diet with a higher omega-3 to omega-6 ratio is more desirable for their overall health (Mount Sinai, n.d.).

Perhaps one of the most common ways to supplement omega-3 fatty acids is with flax seeds. Flax seeds are highly palatable for horses, making them easy to feed. With this said, it is not recommended to feed your horse whole flax seeds. Although not detrimental to your horse's health, the horse's digestive tract is unable to break down the hull of the seed which prevents them from digesting any of the essential fatty acids. So, the best way to feed flax seed is through a stabilized oil form. A cold pressed flax seed oil is best (Crawford, n.d.).

Squash, pumpkins, broccoli, a small amount of collard greens and a small amount of spinach may also be ways to introduce plant-based omega 3 fatty acids into your horse's system (Crawford, n.d.).

Chia seeds provide high quality, digestible fat, 19 of the 20 amino acids, a wide spectrum of vitamins and minerals, and are easy to digest. You can feed chia seeds to horses in their original, virgin form (Mount Sinai, n.d.).

Sainfoin is also referred to as "holy hay." This leafy legume is high in omega-3 fatty acids and offers antimicrobial, anti-parasitic, anti-oxidant, and anti-inflammatory properties (Crawford, n.d.).

Camelina oil, sometimes referred to as false flax oil, is the pressed seed oil of the camelina sativa or false flax plant. Originally used by the ancient Romans for its health benefits, it has recently entered the equine supplement market, due largely in part to its high omega-3 fatty acid profile. It also contains high levels of alpha- and gamma-tocopherol (natural vitamin E). Camelina oil tends to have an earthy smell that many horses find irresistible (Crawford, n.d.).

Hemp oil is naturally rich in omega-3 fatty acids as well as proteins, which can make it a popular supplement for equestrians looking to increase their horse's body condition and/or build muscle. (Crawford, n.d.).

Commonly seen in human omega-3 supplements, fish oil can also be fed to horses to increase their intake of omega-3s. It has been prized for many years for its close ratio of omega-3 to omega-6, while also being very shelf stable. It is important to note that some omega-3 fatty acids derived from fish are not ideal for horses, since fish is not a component of the natural equine diet. (Crawford, n.d.).

Zinc

Zinc is important in respiratory function. It helps the immune system, regenerates cellular damage, and hardens hooves. A deficiency can lead to reduced growth rates, poor performance, lethargy, and rough hair coats (Country Park Herbs, n.d.).

Some common spices and herbs that are high in zinc for your horses include ginger, garlic, turmeric, cumin, oregano, coriander, basil, thyme, paprika, and fennel. Pasture and hay are poor in zinc and horses usually require supplementation with cereal grains such as wheat bran (Team Acko, 2023).

If using a synthetic supplement (not recommended), the minimum requirement for zinc is one and a half teaspoons per day for an adult horse. If your horse is under intense work, just shy of one tablespoon per day is recommended (Quora, n.d.).

Ginseng (Korean or Siberian)

Both types of ginseng support the adrenal glands, which when stressed or exhausted are unable to support the horse's stress functions. No more than one powdered teaspoon daily should be given of the dried powdered root (Suttleworth, 2012).

Echinacea

Echinacea needs to be on-board at the time of any illness. Also, to be effective, one tablespoon of powdered echinacea needs to be given four times a day. You can make it into a tea. Sometimes the horse will drink it straight, but if not, you can add the tea to their water bucket (Wormers-Direct, 2023).

Goldenseal

Goldenseal has antiviral activity and can be given orally by making a tea and adding it to their water bucket or making a tincture. For a horse, thirty to sixty milliliters of a tincture added into their water bucket will help boost their immune system (Fox, n.d.).

Astragalus

Astragalus is used to enhance energy production, which can benefit many organ systems including the lungs, digestion, immune function, cardiac function and even the mind. Three tablespoons of dried and powdered astragalus daily can help with respiratory issues in your horse (Lisa McCann Herb, n.d.).

Garlic

Garlic has been shown in several studies to increase the activity of virus-fighting lymphocytes. If you use garlic in your horse, since it is a "warm" herb in the Chinese pharmacy, make sure you combine it with other herbs that are a bit more cooling, such as mint, elderberry or lemon balm. An average 1,100-pound horse can conservatively consume five teaspoons or five small cloves of garlic per day (The Yale Ledger, 2022).

Turmeric

From the ginger family, this Asian herb is backed by strong data demonstrating its antimicrobial and anti-inflammatory properties (Stronach, 2023).

A dose of **two teaspoons** of powdered turmeric in horses is good for long term use and a dose of one tablespoon per day of turmeric is good for short periods of time (Stronach, 2023).

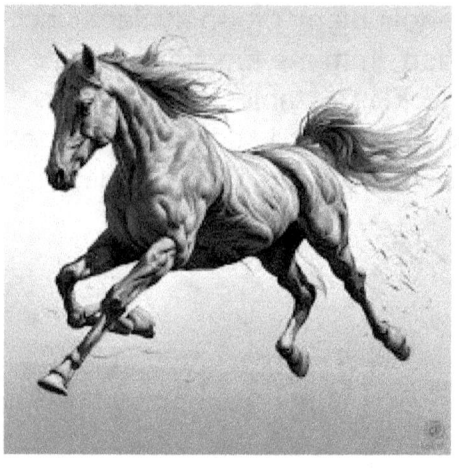

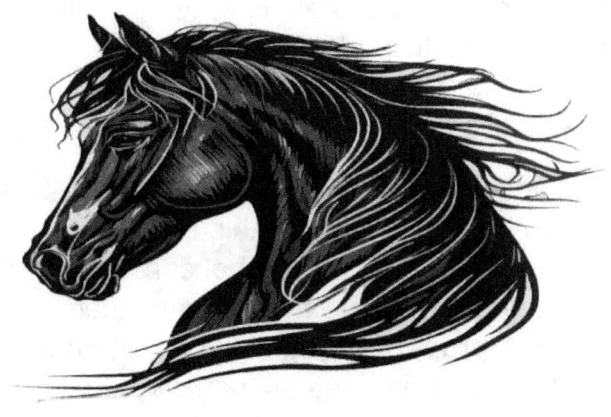

Chapter 7:

General horse information and management

Horses bring a variety of benefits to homesteads, whether by plowing fields, using to haul yourself or other goods from one point to another, or by providing compost for gardens (Homesteaddreamer, 2017).

Horses belong to the family Equidea and includes zebras and donkeys. They can weigh between one thousand five hundred to two thousand two hundred pounds and can be between four and a half to five and a half feet tall, depending on the horse breed (Homesteaddreamer, 2017).

When a baby horse is born, it is called a foal. A male foal up to four years of age is called a colt. Female foals up to four years of age are called fillies (Vedantu, 2023).

After the age of four, a female is called a mare and a male is called a stallion. If a stallion is only used for breeding, that stallion is then called a stud. A gelding is a castrated stallion (Vedantu, 2023).

Like any animal, horses require daily preventative care. I can't stress the importance of this enough. Preventative care is not only herbal care but it also consists of good feed, dry and well-ventilated housing, clean bedding, proper fencing, lots of pasture to exercise, daily grooming, etc. (Spaulding, 2010).

A daily check of your horse is a key part of good care. If you notice any problems, such as lack of appetite, weight loss, diarrhea, constipation, grunting or whining noises, swellings, or other unusual symptoms, give the horse a thorough examination at once. Tomorrow may be too late (Spaulding, 2010).

Check things like teeth, ears, eyes, and feet. Cleaning their teeth will prevent a lot of dental problems that can waste feed, cause infection, and eventually kill a horse (Spaulding, 2010).

Cleaning ears can prevent mites or ticks and discourage bacterial or fungal infections. Checking the horses' eyes are equally important because noticing and treating eye problems right away may save their sight (Spaulding, 2010).

The horse's feet should not be overlooked. It's a lot easier to clean a horse's hooves regularly than to deal with the devastating effects of thrush. Same can be said for a stone in the horse's hoof....after it has caused severe pain, bruising, or infection, treatment can be a lengthy and frustrating process (Spaulding, 2010).

With any type of animal, you will have to face a health concern at some point. The best way is to prevent that health concern from happening is by staying on top of what your horse really needs; however, sometimes ailments happen whether there were prevention protocols in place or not. Regular attention, good general care, and routine checkups are the keys to healthy horses and happy animal owners (Spaulding, 2010).

Space

In some areas, two acres of land is adequate. In other areas, one hundred acres may not be enough to provide sufficient grazing. A horse should not eat the pasture to the ground. If they do, the grazing area is limited of nutrients and you must supplement them with good quality hay (Spaulding, 2010).

Foaling

The gestation period of a horse is eleven months. This means from the time of conception to the time the baby is delivered, there is eleven months (Spaulding, 2010).

Most horse's labor and delivery are in the early morning or late at night and only lasts about fifteen to twenty minutes. Before they give birth, the mare may pace, isolates herself to a corner, sweat, and most often will lie down to deliver (Spaulding, 2010).

Exercise

Just like with humans, horses need exercise. Movement and breathing in good air with a bit of sunshine on the face can do a body good. Even a pregnant mare needs daily exercise. Exercise helps keep weight off and weight on a horse can cause a lot of health issues. Movement can also keep joint stiffness and pain to a minimum (Spaulding, 2010).

Body Temperature

What kind of thermometer should I use? There are two types available. A mercury bulb thermometer is inexpensive but easily broken. There are also electronic thermometers which are a bit more expensive but they last longer and are easier to read (Spaulding, 2010).

The basic thermometers found on the market for humans can do the job with some finagling; however, they do make longer probe thermometers specifically for livestock animals. It is also helpful, but not necessary, to have the disposable plastic sheaths that go over the thermometer so that if any fecal matter gets on the thermometer, its easily removed when the plastic sheath is taken off.

The technique needed to find out your horse's body temperature is as follows: Stand close to left hand side of the horse to avoid being kicked. Make sure the horse knows you are there. Lubricate the end of the thermometer with soapy water, lubricant, or soothing salve. Move the tail to the side (PennState Extension, 2023).

If using a mercury thermometer gently shake the mercury down to the bottom of the tube. Lift the tail and gently insert the thermometer into the horse's rectum. Make sure the tip of the thermometer rests against the rectal wall and not into a clump of manure (PennState Extension, 2023).

Hold the end of the thermometer tightly to stop it from disappearing up the rectum. If you are using a mercury thermometer wait at least sixty seconds before removing the thermometer and reading it. Electronic thermometers will 'beep' when an accurate reading is obtained (PennState Extension, 2023).

An adult horse at rest should have a body temperature of 99 - 101.5 degrees Fahrenheit. Anything above that level can indicate an active infection. The normal temperature range for a foal is 99.5 - 102.1 degrees Fahrenheit (Lentz, n.d.).

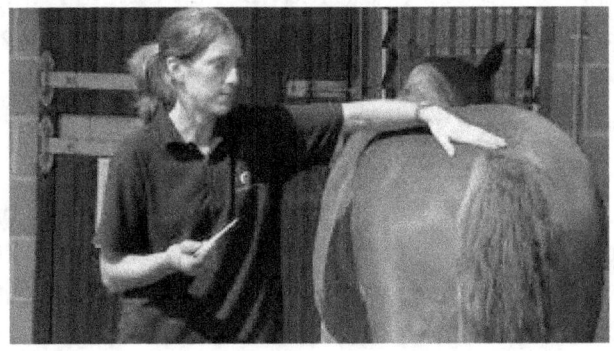

Hooves

Good hoof care is a vital part of keeping your horse healthy. If the horse is kept in a stall daily, they need their feet cleaned daily. Without this, stabled horses' hooves can become packed with manure which can lead to thrush (Spaulding, 2010).

Hooves normally grow out and require regular trimming. Some horses will have brittle hooves. They usually have a tendency to develop cracks, splits, and chips. These issues can then lead to other serious health concerns (Spaulding, 2010).

Toxic plants to horses

Plants that are toxic to horses aren't particularly rare. Take a stroll through any pasture, and there among the grasses you'll find any number of different plants both medicinal and toxic. Small vines, broad-leafed weeds, some wildflowers you might recognize—some you won't. As disquieting as it may be to contemplate, the chances are pretty good that at least some are toxic to horses. Hundreds of poisonous plants grow in North America, and many are extremely common (Equus Magazine, 2022).

The good news, of course, is that the vast majority of those plants pose little threat to horses. For one thing, most of them are unpalatable, and horses who are filling up on quality forage aren't likely to spend a lot of time grazing on the few bitter leaves populating their pasture (Equus Magazine, 2022).

Remember how I mentioned that animals have an innate ability to know what plants they need and what plants they do not, also known as Zoopharmacognosy?. Unless your animal is starving, they will most likely avoid toxic plants and just eat plants that are healthy for them.

Another factor that protects horses is their size. A one-thousand-pound animal has to consume significantly higher quantities of most toxins than a smaller animal does to feel any effects. So, for the most part, as long as your horses are healthy and your pasture is in good shape, you have little to worry about (Equus Magazine, 2022).

However, some plants are cause for concern either because even a curious nibble can spell doom or because repeated browsing over weeks or months can lead to serious illness and death. All are worth getting to know by sight—not only so you can eliminate them from your horse keeping areas, but also so that you can avoid encounters with them in the woods, on the roadsides, and along the paths where you ride. This is NOT a complete list; however, this list can help guide you.

Black Walnut (Juglans Nigra)

Black walnut is a tall tree valued for its decorative wood. It grows to be about sixty-five to one hundred feet tall and has a trunk about two to three feet in diameter. The roots of black walnut exude chemicals called juglones that can inhibit the growth of other plants and be toxic to some animals (Britannica, n.d.).

Horses may be affected by black walnut chips or sawdust when they are used for bedding material. Close association with walnut trees while pollen is being shed (typically in May) also produce allergic symptoms in both horses and humans. The juglone toxin occurs in the leaves, bark and wood of walnut, but these contain lower concentrations than in the roots (Funt, n.d.).

Bracken fern *(Pteridum aquilinum)*

Bracken fern is a perennial fern with triangular leaves that can reach two to three feet high. It grows in clumps in woodlands and moist open areas (PennState Extension, 2023).

Bracken fern contains thiaminase, which inhibits absorption of thiamin, which is vitamin B1. Thiamin is necessary to nerve function, and deficiencies can lead to neurological impairment, depression, incoordination, and blindness. The relative toxicity of individual leaves is low—horses must consume hundreds of pounds to experience ill effects. However, bracken fern is unique among the toxic plants in that some horses seem to develop a taste for it and will seek it out even when other forages are available (PennState Extension, 2023).

Hemlock *(Conium maculatum)*

Hemlock is a multi-stemmed perennial weed with toothed, fernlike leaves and clusters of small white flowers. The stems have purple spots, which are most evident near the base of the plant. It grows wild along roadsides and other open uncultivated areas throughout North America. This hemlock is commonly referred to as 'poison hemlock' and is not to be confused with the tree, also commonly called hemlock *(Tsuga)*, within the pine family (PennState Extension, 2023).

Hemlock leaves, stems and seeds contain several potent neurotoxins that affect both the central and peripheral nervous systems. Four to five pounds is a lethal dose for a horse. Most animals will avoid the plant. Signs appear within an hour or two of consumption, starting with nervousness, tremors and incoordination, progressing to depression and diminished heart and respiratory rates and possibly colic. Death results from respiratory failure (Garland, n.d.).

Tansy ragwort (Senecio spp.)

Tansy ragwort is a multi-stemmed weed with alternating leaves that produces clusters of small daisy-like yellow flowers. It is commonly seen in pastures and along roadsides (PennState Extension, 2023).

Levels of toxicity vary among different members of the species, but all are thought to contain at least some concentration of pyrrolizidine alkaloids, which inhibit cell division, especially in the liver. Damage to the liver is cumulative and irreversible, and most horses succumb to chronic exposure over time, after consuming between fifty and one hundred and fifty pounds, in total. Signs include diminished appetite and weight loss, depression, incoordination, and jaundice (PennState Extension, 2023).

~~~~~~

Johnsongrass/Sudan grass (*Sorghum* spp.)

Both Johnsongrass and Sudan grass are coarse-stemmed grasses with broad, veined leaves that can grow to six feet in height. Both produce large, multibranched seed heads (PennState Extension, 2023).

Johnsongrass is a wild grass native to the southern climates, where it grows along roadways and other uncultivated open areas. A close relative, Sudan grass, and its hybrids are cultivated throughout the United States as a forage crop (PennState Extension, 2023).

The leaves and stems of johnsongrass/sudan grass contain a cyanide compound, which when metabolized inhibits the body's ability to absorb oxygen, in effect suffocating the animal; young shoots of johnsongrass contain the highest concentration of the toxin. Because horses do not metabolize the cyanide compound as efficiently as ruminant animals do, grazing plants is likely to harm them (PennState Extension, 2023).

Cultivated hybrids of Sudan grass typically contain less cyanide, if any. Both species can also accumulate toxic levels of nitrates if overfertilized. Cyanide concentration drops to safe levels when the grasses are cured for hay, but nitrates, if present, do not (PennState Extension, 2023).

Signs of poisoning include rapid breathing, which progresses to tremors, frequent urination and defecation, gasping, and convulsions (PennState Extension, 2023).

~~~~~~

Locoweed (*Astragalus* spp. or *Oxytropis* spp.)

Locoweed is a leafy perennial with short stems and compound leaves that grow in tuftlike forms from a single taproot. There are many different species. Some species may be covered with silvery hairs. The flowers, often white or purple, are borne on leafless stalks. They grow in varied terrains throughout the West and Southwest, often in dry, sandy soil (PennState Extension, 2023).

All toxic species of locoweed contain swainsonine, an alkaloid that inhibits the production of the enzyme necessary for saccharaide metabolism, and the resulting sugar buildup disrupts the function of brain cells (PennState Extension, 2023).

Strange behavior is usually the first evidence noticed; horses may bob their heads, adopt exaggerated, high-stepping gaits, or stagger and fall (PennState Extension, 2023).

Oleander *(Nerium oleander)*

Oleander, also known as rose laurel, is an evergreen shrub that can reach the size of a small tree. It has elongated, thick leathery leaves that can grow to three to ten inches long. The flowers, which grow in large clusters at the end of branches, are one to three inches in diameter and can be white, pink or red (PennState Extension, 2023).

All parts of the plant contain the toxins oleandrin and neriin, which disrupt the beating of the heart. The leaves remain toxic when dried. About 30 to 40 leaves can be deadly to a horse (PennState Extension, 2023).

Signs that your horse has ingested Oleander include colic, difficulty breathing, tremors, recumbency, and an irregular heart rate. The pulse may be either slowed or accelerated. Effects are usually seen several hours after ingestion and last over twenty-four hours. Administration of activated charcoal can help if treated immediately after ingestion (PennState Extension, 2023).

Red maple trees *(Acer rubrum)*

Red maple trees are medium-sized with leaves that are green in the spring and summer. They have shallow notches, bright red stems and a whitish underside; in fall, the leaves turn bright red. The bark is smooth and pale gray on young trees, and becomes dark and broken on older trees (PennState Extension, 2023).

The ingestion of fresh, growing red maple leaves seems to do little or no harm, but when the leaves wilt, they become extremely toxic to horses. Access to wilted leaves is most common after storms, which may cause branches to fall into pastures, or in the autumn when the leaves fall and are blown into grazing areas. The toxins in wilted red maple leaves cause the red blood cells to break down so that the blood can no longer carry oxygen; the kidneys, liver and other organs may also be damaged. As little as a pound or two of leaves can be fatal (PennState Extension, 2023).

Depending on how many leaves were eaten, signs can appear within a few hours or as long as four or five days after consumption. They include lethargy, refusal to eat, dark red-brown or black urine, discolored gums (pale yellowish gums at first, advancing to dark muddy brown), increased respiratory rate, rapid heart rate, and dehydration (PennState Extension, 2023).

Please note that the leaves of the silver and sugar maples may contain the same toxic elements as red maples, but in less toxic amounts (PennState Extension, 2023).

<u>Water hemlock</u> (*Cicuta* spp.)

Water hemlock, also known as false parsley, is a perennial weed with erect hairless stems that can grow to six feet from clusters of fleshy roots. The stems are hollow and branching, thicker at the base. Leaves are elongated and toothed, and the small white flowers form flat, umbrella-shaped clusters at the ends of branches (PennState Extension, 2023).

Water hemlock is considered one of the most toxic plants in the United States. All parts of the plant contain a cicutoxin alkaloid that affects the central nervous system, but the toxin is most concentrated in the root. Because cattle are more likely to pull up and consume the root, that species is considered most at risk of poisoning, but horses have also been known to browse the plant; less than a pound of the leaves and stems can be fatal. The toxin levels in the leaves and stems diminish as the plant ages during the growing season, and additional amounts of toxin are lost when the plant is dried, but water hemlock is never considered safe for consumption. Most animals will avoid the plant (PennState Extension, 2023).

The toxins affect neurons primarily within the brain, causing various signs, including excessive salivation, dilated pupils and nervousness, progressing rapidly to difficult breathing, degeneration of the heart and skeletal muscles, seizures and convulsions; death usually results from respiratory paralysis. Signs of poisoning appear within an hour of ingestion, and death typically follows within two to three hours (PennState Extension, 2023).

Yellow star thistle/Russian knapweed (*Centauria* spp.)

Yellow star thistle is an annual weed that branches out from a single base stem to form a spherical plant up to three feet tall; its round yellow flowers are surrounded by stiff spines 1/2 to 3/4 of an inch long. Russian knapweed spreads via a creeping root system; its erect, stiff stems grow two to three feet high and are covered with gray hairs, and its thistlelike flowers range from purple to white; Russian knapweed has no spines or prickles (PennState Extension, 2023).

Both plants contain a toxic agent that has a neurological effect on the brain that inhibits the nerves and controls chewing. The poisoning is chronic in nature; to receive a toxic dose, horses must consume fifty to two hundred percent of their body weight over thirty to ninety days (PennState Extension, 2023).

Affected horses may appear to have tense or clenched facial muscles, and they are unable to bite or chew their food effectively. Weight loss is also common (PennState Extension, 2023).

Yew (*Taxus* spp.)

Yew is a woody evergreen shrub with closely spaced, flat, needlelike leaves a half-inch to one inch long. Berries are bright red or yellow, soft and juicy with a hole in the end, where the dark seed is visible (PennState Extension, 2023).

All parts of the yew plant, except for the fleshy portion of the berries, contain taxine, an alkaloid that causes respiratory and cardiac collapse. The leaves remain toxic even after dried. A single mouthful can be deadly to a horse within minutes (PennState Extension, 2023).

Sudden death is the most typical sign of yew ingestion. Animals found alive may be trembling and colicky, with difficulty breathing and a slowed heart rate (PennState Extension, 2023).

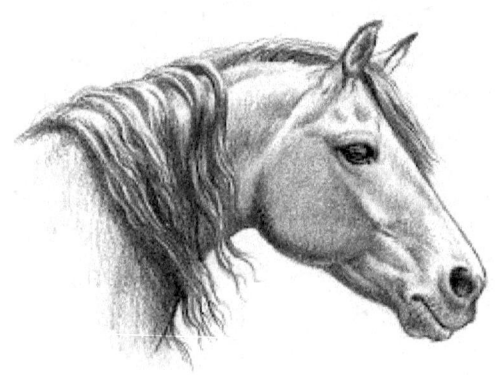

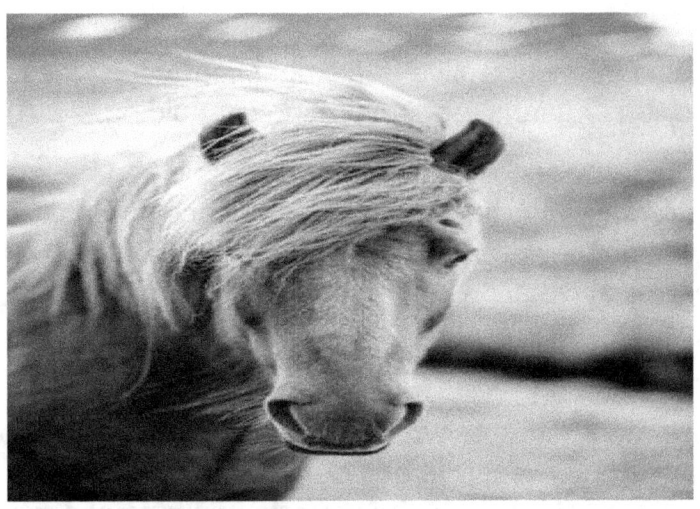

Chapter 8:

Horse Ailments/problems/health concerns

While horses are generally quite hardy and disease-free, it is smart to be aware of health problems that might happen.

Let's take a look at some common horse health (equine) concerns. Any dosing mentioned is based on an 1100-pound horse (with the exception of foul pneumonia)

COLIC

Colic is one of the most common gastrointestinal problems occurring in horses. It affects horses more so than other mammals. This extremely painful abdominal condition can be caused by untreated dental issues, not having enough roughage in their diet, excessive gas accumulation in the colon, accumulation of indigestible material in the digestive tract, ingestion of parasites, ingestion of sands, or dehydration (Spaulding, 2010).

The severity of colic can vary greatly and can be fatal if left untreated. A horse that is experiencing the pain of colic might paw, roll, and have trouble defecating. They may also have a loss of appetite, lack normal gut sounds, sweat, have an increased heart rate, or have an urge to constantly urinate (Spaulding, 2010).

There are 3 different types of colic in horses. Gas colic is caused by excessive gas buildup in the horse's digestive system. This can cause symptoms of stress and abdominal pain in your horse. Gas colic is thought to commonly be caused by a sudden change in a horse's feed (Spaulding, 2010).

Another type of colic in horses is impaction colic. This form of colic is marked by gastrointestinal distress caused by physical obstruction of the digestive system. These blockages are often caused by hardened dry clumps of food but can also be caused if your horse consumes a foreign object. Sand or dirt are common examples of foreign materials that can potentially cause impaction colic (Spaulding, 2010).

The third type of colic in horses is spasmodic colic. Spasmodic colic occurs when the stomach and digestive system muscles contract, causing pain and difficulties defecating. It is commonly caused by stress, similar to common indigestion in humans. Spasmodic colic can often be effectively treated by a veterinarian (Spaulding, 2010).

PREVENTION

Colic is a serious affliction for horses that can have fatal consequences if left untreated. As such, horse owners can take a sigh of relief in knowing there are ways they can potentially reduce the risk of their horse's developing colic. There is no one way to ensure that your horses are not at risk for it, but with consistent care practices, checking your horse's vital signs, and maintenance using natural processes, you can minimize the risk of your horse developing colic (Holistapet, n.d.).

One of the easiest home remedies for colic is a good diet! Horses prone to colic can benefit from a dietary overhaul. In the wild, horses graze and feed on low-energy plants such as grass for as long as twelve hours at a time. Modern feeding methods do not account for this and, as a result, often do not provide everything a horse needs to avoid digestive problems. Modern feeding regimens also lack the proper spacing between meals, nutritional density, and portions to prevent your horse's digestive tract problems (Holistapet, n.d.).

One simple method for creating a proper feeding regimen for your horse is to feed them only what they need. Overfeeding can reduce gut motility and lead to a case of equine colic if left unchecked. Feed them simple grass. It will help stimulate gut motility by providing it with consistent balanced gut activity. Consistent gut activity is a major way to reduce colic risk because a horse's digestive system has evolved to constantly digest and process food (Holistapet, n.d.).

TREATMENT

Herbal remedies to help horses with colic include dandelion, chamomile, valerian root, meadowsweet herb, and peppermint (Brookby Herbs, 2018). Dandelion is full of vitamins and minerals including calcium, iron, potassium, and beta carotene which can help boost digestion and relieve an upset stomach. Just mix two cups of this fresh or dried herb into their feed (ESC, n.d.)

Chamomile is known for its anti-inflammatory properties. It also promotes relaxation in the body which can aid in the digestive process. This can be beneficial for any horse experiencing colic. Horses also tend to prefer the taste of chamomile so it is easy to add the one forth a cup fresh or powdered chamomile to their feed two times a day (Brookby Herbs, 2018).

While valerian root is used as a sedative for humans, it can be used to promote relaxation in horses. This can be helpful for digestion and gastric discomfort. It is commonly used to treat mild colic symptoms in horses. You can add one tablespoon powdered valerian root to their feed; however, a decoction tea may also help. Just add this tea into their normal water bucket (Brookby Herbs, 2018).

Meadowsweet herb has effects similar to aspirin. Because it possesses anti-inflammatory properties, it can help with equine arthritis as well as gut problems. Add two teaspoons of this fresh or powdered herb into their feed twice a day or you can make a tea and add this into their water bucket (ESC, n.d.).

Peppermint is known to aid in the digestive process and help relieve pain caused by colic. To administer this, simply mix some peppermint leaves into their feed to help your horse's digestive system or use one tablespoon of powdered peppermint in their feed. Also, peppermint essential oil can be used topically. Apply around twenty drops to the horse's abdomen to provide soothing relief (Brookby Herbs, 2018).

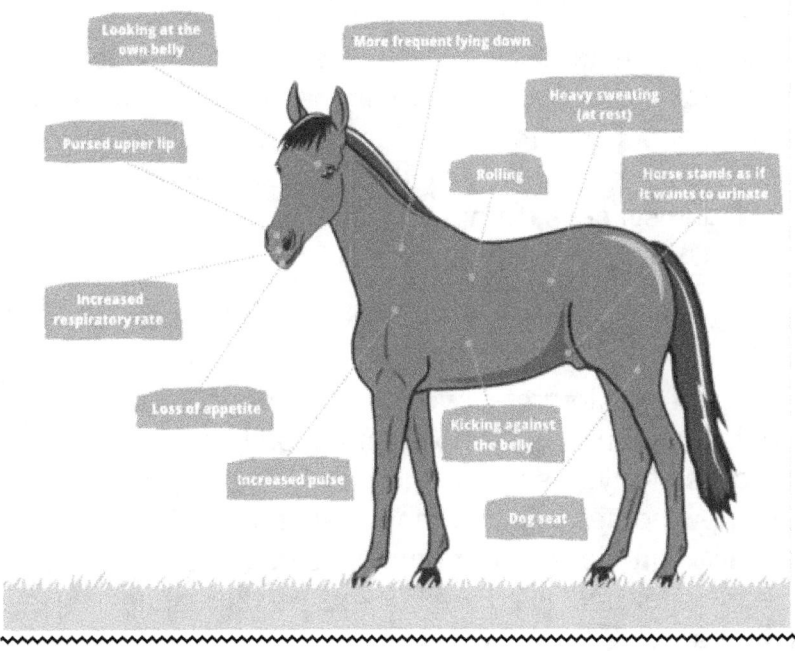

EQUINE INFLUENZA (FLU)

Equine influenza is an acute, highly contagious, viral disease which can cause rapidly spreading outbreaks of respiratory disease in horses and other equine species (Spaulding, 2010).

Humans do not get infected with equine influenza. However, humans can physically carry the virus on their skin, hair, clothing and shoes, and can therefore transfer the virus to other horses (Spaulding, 2010).

The main signs that your horse may have equine influenza is a sudden increase in temperature, a deep, dry, hacking cough; and a watery nasal discharge, which may later become mucopurulent. Other signs can include depression, loss of appetite, labored breathing, muscle pain, and stiffness (Spaulding, 2010).

PREVENTION

The best way to protect your horse from contracting equine influenza is to implement good hygiene practices for yourself and the horse. Also, quarantine any new horses in a different location for at least twenty-eight days. Your horse should have their own clean water buckets, feed buckets, and brushes (Chahan, 2022).

TREATMENT

Treatment for equine influenza involves treating with herbs and allowing your horse to rest. Just like the human flu virus, there is no cure for equine influenza.

At least six weeks of rest are recommended in order for the damaged liner of the upper respiratory tract to adequately heal (Argyle Veterinary Hospital, n.d.).

While your horse is healing, they should be stabled in a clean, well-ventilated area to avoid excess dust, which may exasperate their condition further. They should also be supplied with plenty of fresh hay, herbs, and water. Sometimes horses can develop secondary infections, such as pneumonia, from equine influenza (Heeringa, 2023).

Herbal treatments include tulsi basil and echinacea. Tulsi basil is a holy plant with medicinal properties. It has been known for its medicinal effects on viral infections. Tulsi (Holy basil) has antimicrobial, anti-inflammatory, anti-allergic, and many more medicinal properties. Tulsi basil has immunity-enhancing properties that help the body fight against every type of infectious bacteria and virus. It has anti-allergic properties that will facilitate easy recovery from equine influenza. Four powdered tablespoons daily will increase the overall immunity that will regain the stamina of the horses (Spaulding, 2010).

Boosting your horse's immune system is crucial when they have equine influenza. Boosting it naturally can be as simple as adding four powdered tablespoons daily of echinacea into their diet. Echinacea has purple or white flowers, which grows to approximately three feet tall. It is also known as coneflower for its conic-shaped flowers and has been used for centuries for humans and animals as a treatment for colds, flu, and general infections (Equalite Herbals, 2020). (See chapter 6: Immune System)

You can also aid in the horse's respiratory system by adding a few of the following herbs.

Coltsfoot leaves, (Tussilago farfara) known historically as the "cough plant," can have anti-inflammatory, anti-spasmodic and anti-catarrhal (eases inflammation of mucous membranes) properties. Two powdered tablespoons daily can be useful for respiratory tract disorders in 1100-pound horses, particularly to relieve coughing (Spaulding, 2010).

Elder flowers (Sambucas nigra) Have been used throughout history for upper respiratory tract infections and are widely reported to be beneficial for colds and flu. Elder is a pungent, cooling herb that can have anti-catarrhal and anti-inflammatory effects, making it useful for respiratory tract disorders. The berries are toxic if eaten raw, however about a cup of elder flowers daily can be fed to an average 1100-pound horse safely (Spaulding, 2010).

Comfrey helps with respiratory problems in horses. Forty leaves for an average 1100-pound horse can be given daily to aid with congested lungs and other respiratory issues. Another herb that is similar to Comfrey is Houndstongue. It can be given at the same ratio (Mount Sinai, n.d.).

Elecampane or Culver's Root is widely used as an expectorant and cough suppressant. The herb also has anti-bacterial properties that can protect the sinus and guttural pouch from infections. Dosing is one half to one teaspoon of powdered root, four times a day for an average 1100-pound horse (The Plaid Horse, 2021).

Eyebright (Euphrasia officinalis) is a small annual herb native to Europe. The flowering eyebright herb has been used since the middle-ages as a bronchial dilator. Eyebright should not be fed to breeding stallions. The daily dose of two tablespoons powdered eyebright for an average 1100-pound horse is sufficient (Horse Herbs, n.d.).

Fenugreek, also known as Bird's Foot, is distilled from the dried ripe seeds of the plant and has anti-inflammatory and anti-fungal properties that can reduce the production of thick mucus. For an average 1100-pound horse, one teaspoon to two tablespoons of powdered Fenugreek can be given to your horse daily (Smartpak, n.d.).

Garlic is pungent herb with antimicrobial, expectorant, anti-inflammatory, and antioxidant properties. All these make it a good choice for respiratory disorders. Five small cloves of garlic per day per an average 1100-pound horse should do the trick (NSW Government, n.d.).

Mullein is a good lung herb to strengthen weakened tissue and to help horses breathe easier. Mullein is a biennial herb which means it has a two-year lifespan. In the second year, mullein will flower and is the best time for harvesting. The flowers and leaves are the medicinal part that is good for horses especially if paired with yarrow, elecampane herb, or lungwort herb (Honeyvale Herbs, n.d.)

RHINOPNEUMONITIS/EQUINE HERPESVIRUS (EHV)

Rhinopneumonitis, also known as equine herpesvirus, is a highly infectious virus found virtually worldwide. There are currently nine known EHVs. EHV-1, EHV-3, and EHV-4 pose the highest disease risk in the U.S. horse population. EHV-1 and EHV-4 can cause upper respiratory disease, neurological disease, abortions, and/or neonatal death. EHV-3 causes a venereal disease called coital exanthema. In recent years there has been an increase in the number of EHV-1 neurologic cases, also referred to as Equine Herpes Myeloencephalopathy (EHM). The virus incubation period is highly variable and can be as long as fourteen days. Prognosis is good for horses not affected with the neurologic form and varies for those with neurologic signs (Spaulding, 2010).

Initial symptoms may be vague – fever, lack of appetite, and lethargy – and can progress rapidly to the neurologic form.

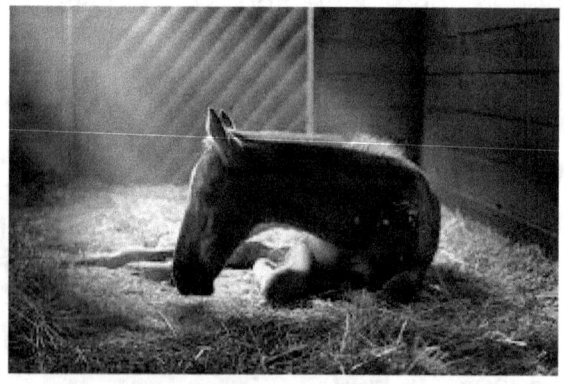

Neurological symptoms include incoordination, leaning against walls for stability, urinary incontinence or dribbling, loss of tail tone, paralysis, and eventually an inability to stand (Spaulding, 2010).

PREVENTION

Vaccines are available to prevent the respiratory and abortion forms of EHV, however I'm not one who feels vaccines are needed. When there are ways to prevent diseases naturally, why not do that rather than putting toxic manmade medication into an animal? Vaccines were not around hundreds of years ago and horses survived. If they had not, they would not be here today. If you do decide to go the vaccine route, there are none labeled as effective against the neurologic form of the disease (Spaulding, 2010).

In general, vaccinating in the face of an outbreak is always controversial. It has been demonstrated that many vaccinations can cause a transitory period of immune-suppression, so an animal could be at greater risk if exposed during that period. Also, the intramuscular vaccines usually require at least one week for measurable humoral responses to a booster or a second dose. This time lag discourages the effectiveness of the vaccine (Spaulding, 2010).

TREATMENT

The horses own immune system is still the best protection. In the face of environmental or performance stresses, immune support may delay, decrease, or prevent clinical signs. To support immune function, try to avoid alterations to the horse's gut microbiome (pharmaceutical and suppressive medications) and also avoid things that can suppress the immune system, such as stress from travel, strange places, and separation from herd buddies (Homegrown Herbalist, n.d.)

Stimulate and support the immune system function with nutrition and herbs. Using nutrition to boost immunity involves feeding whole, clean, quality grains but be cautious using overly processed feeds with ingredients made from by-products, since these actually increase oxidative stress in the body (Homegrown Herbalist, n.d.) (See Chapter 6: Immune System)

Comfrey leaves have been shown to help with respiratory issues in horses. Forty leaves daily for an average 1100-pound horse will help (Homegrown Herbalist, n.d.).

Three tablespoons daily of astragalus has also been shown to help with rhinopneumonitis/equine herpesvirus (EHV) especially when mixed with Ligustrum. Ligustrum is an evergreen shrub, also known as Chinese Privet, that should be given in very small amounts. Large amounts in a horse can cause staggering, diarrhea, convulsions, and/or paralysis. Never do more than a half teaspoon daily for more than three days concurrently (McDowell's, n.d.).

EQUINE ENCEPHALOMYELITIS (Sleeping Sickness)

Equine encephalomyelitis, often referred to as "sleeping sickness," is a concerning infectious disease that primarily affects the horse's brain. This can affect humans as well. This ailment is caused by a virus and categorized into three distinct strains. Those strains are Eastern, Western, and Venezuelan strains. They each carry varying degrees of mortality risk. Among these strains, the Eastern variant is both the most prevalent and the most lethal (Young, 2020).

The transmission of encephalomyelitis is facilitated by a network of organisms. The virus finds its home in reservoir hosts, which include birds, reptiles, and rodents. These reservoir hosts are a key part of the virus's life cycle. Mosquitoes, acting as vectors, play a crucial role by transferring the virus from these reservoir hosts to horses. Consequently, the disease tends to manifest most prominently from midsummer until the arrival of frost. It's important to note that while horses can transmit the disease to one another through close contact, such as rubbing noses or sharing feed and water containers, they are regarded as "dead-end hosts" due to their low viral count. This makes it highly unlikely for feeding mosquitoes to contract the virus from infected horses (Spaulding, 2010).

Signs of encephalomyelitis in your horse can include fever, depression, gastrointestinal distress, altered mental state, behavior changes, and central nervous system symptoms. These symptoms can typically look like one or more of the following; a general sense of lethargy, diarrhea, drowsy appearance, lack of interest to move around, self-mutilation, hyperexcitability, irritability, refusal of food and water, incoordination, head pressing, circling, paralysis, convulsions, and/or coma. Unfortunately, death typically occurs within two to three days after the initial signs appear (**Spaulding, 2010**).

PREVENTION

Western medicine will highly recommend a series of two vaccinations as the best way to prevent this disease. While it can help to administer before mosquito season begins in the spring or early summer and the second dosage two to four weeks later, the immunity will only last approximately six months and any vaccine administered will lower the horse's immune system. The best way to prevent this naturally is reducing mosquito populations around horse facilities. Employing mosquito control measures, such as eliminating breeding sites and using mosquito repellents, can be effective in mitigating the risk. Herbal mosquito repellents that can be planted around your horse keeping area include marigolds, catnip, citronella, basil, lavender, rosemary, peppermint, geranium, lemon balm, and garlic. Make sure your horse can not reach these to eat as some are toxic to horses such as catnip and citronella (**Apfel, 2018**).

TREATMENT

There is no cure for equine encephalitis with either pharmaceutical medication or herbal medication. Treatment largely consists of keeping the horse comfortable, either through anti-inflammatory pharmaceuticals and intravenous fluids or three to four tablespoons (divided and given in two separate meals) of white willow bark. Aspirin may cause stomach ulcerations whereas white willow bark is gentler on the stomach. It contains salicin which helps reduce body temperature and inflammation (Texas Horseman, 2023).

Other safe and useful anti-inflammatory herbs consist of one teaspoon of powdered boswellia twice a day, one teaspoon powdered devil's claw per day (harpagophytum procumbens only), four tablespoons powdered nettle leaves, two teaspoons of celery seed per day, three to four tablespoons of rose hips daily, and one tablespoon of powdered turmeric daily. With the devil's claw, it could increase gastric juices and therefore should not be given to a horse with a history of gastric ulcers (Equus Vitalis, n.d.).

It is important to note that the 'sleeping sickness' will make your horse need to lay down for extended periods of time. Because of this, bedsores could arise so it is best to rotate the horse periodically (Texas Horseman, 2023).

EQUINE INFECTIOUS ANEMIA VIRUS (EIA)

Equine Infectious Anemia (EIA) is a viral disease found widely throughout the world. Horse flies and deer flies can transmit equine infectious anemia. It is can be transmitted to foals in utero and sometimes via milk or semen (USDA, 2023).

If the horse survives the acute phase of the infection, they will carry this disease with them, making them contagious to other horses throughout their lifetime. Because of this, they must be permanently quarantined or euthanized. If the horse is permanently quarantined, it can have recurrent flare-ups if their stress load is too much (USDA, 2023).

Signs for equine infectious anemia are often nonspecific and of variable severity. The signs can range from fever and decreased appetite to severe anemia and sudden death. It is often difficult to differentiate equine infectious anemia from other diseases. Incubation period is a one week to eight weeks or longer. Additional signs in an acute case can include jaundice, rapid breathing, rapid heart rate, swelling of limbs, bleeding from the nose, red/purple spots on mucous membranes, or blood-stained feces (USDA, 2023).

If you suspect equine infectious anemia, move the horse at least six hundred feet away from other horses and try to reduce exposure to horse and/or deer flies (USDA, 2023).

PREVENTION

Observation and horse/deer fly repellants are the two best methods of prevention.

Herbal horse fly and deer fly repellents that can be planted around your horse keeping area include marigolds, catnip, citronella, basil, lavender, rosemary, peppermint, geranium, lemon balm, garlic, lemon grass, tansy, sage, bay laurel, bay leaves, thyme, eucalyptus, chives, borage, chrysanthemum, yarrow, oregano, allium, bee balm, and wormwood. Make sure your horse can not reach these to eat as some are toxic to horses such as catnip and citronella (Spaulding, 2010).

TREATMENT

There is no treatment for equine infectious anemia. If the owner chooses not to euthanize, the quarantined horse needs a stress-free environment away from strenuous work and avoiding other illnesses. Boosting their immune system with herbs may be your only course of action. Those immune boosting herbs are one teaspoon powdered Korean or Siberian Ginseng per day, one tablespoon powdered echinacea, three tablespoons powdered astragalus daily, five small cloves garlic per day, and two teaspoons powdered turmeric per day (Immubiom, 2021). (See chapter 6: Immune System)

WEST NILE VIRUS

West Nile Virus (WNV) is a viral disease that can result in fever, incoordination, hind-end weakness, depression, anorexia, muscle tremors, teeth grinding, inability to swallow, head pressing, excessive sweating, behavior changes, neurologic problems, and inability to rise from the ground.   These signs usually present within about fifteen days after a bite from an infected mosquito (Spaulding, 2010).

The virus was introduced to the United States in 1999. Since then, over twenty-seven thousand horses have been infected and the west nile virus is considered an endemic disease (Spaulding, 2010).

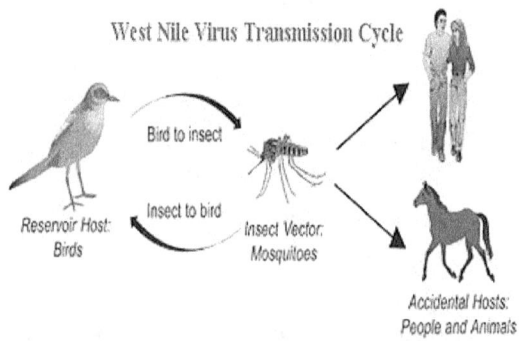

West Nile Virus Transmission Cycle

Bird to insect

Insect to bird

Reservoir Host:
Birds

Insect Vector:
Mosquitoes

Accidental Hosts:
People and Animals

The west nile virus is transmitted by infected mosquitoes. Wild birds serve as the host reservoir. When mosquitos feed on infected birds, they become infected and can transmit the virus to other birds, horses, and even humans (Spaulding, 2010).

PREVENTION

An herbal oil or herbal tea can be made and put on the horse topically. In either of these, use lemongrass, cedarwood, geranium, and rosemary. If making an herbal oil, make sure the oil you use is safe for horses (USDA, 2022)

Minimize mosquito habitats by removing any standing or stagnant water where mosquitos may be hatching their eggs. You also need to maintain very clean stalls and use stall fans (USDA, 2022).

In addition, plant mosquito repellent herbs around your horse keeping area. These herbs include marigolds, catnip, citronella, basil, lavender, rosemary, peppermint, geranium, lemon balm, and garlic. Make sure your horse can not reach these to eat as some are toxic to horses such as catnip and citronella (USDA, 2022).

TREATMENT

Treatment consists of boosting the immune system as much as possible with herbs such as three tablespoons powdered astragalus per day, five teaspoons of garlic per day (about five cloves), two tablespoons powdered turmeric per day, one teaspoon of powdered ginseng per day, six to twelve teaspoons tincture of goldenseal daily, and one tablespoon powdered echinacea three times a day. (See chapter 6: Immune System). Prognosis may be poor for horses with severe neurologic signs. The west nile virus mortality rate is about thirty-five percent (USDA, 2022).

It would also be a good idea to add three and a half tablespoons of powdered Tulsi (holy) basil daily. Tulsi has immunity-enhancing properties that help the body fight against every type of infectious bacteria and virus. It has anti-allergic properties that will facilitate easy recovery from an equine illness (USDA, 2022).

STREPTOCOCCUS EQUI (Strangles)

Streptococcus equi, or 'strangles' is a highly contagious bacterial disease seen worldwide caused by Streptococcus equi equi. It is the most common infection in horses ages six to ten (Spaulding, 2010).

Horses become infected through inhalation or ingestion of the equi equi bacteria. The bacteria crosses the mucous membranes in the nose and mouth to infect the lymph nodes. In the lymph nodes, abscesses rupture and the infected lymph nodes become swollen which can compress the upper respiratory tract. It can occur through horse-to-horse contact, drinking contaminated water, or making contact with infected equipment or clothing (Spaulding, 2010).

Although some horses may not show signs or symptoms, they can carry this bacteria to other horses. There is an incubation period of three to eight days at which time the usual signs include lethargy, anorexia, sudden onset fever of greater than 103 degrees Fahrenheit, nasal discharge, swelling of the lymph nodes, and the formation of abscesses, primarily in the head and neck. Disease severity varies and younger horses often exhibit more severe signs than older horses (Spaulding, 2010).

The prognosis of uncomplicated cases is good and usually takes three to six weeks. Disease severity varies and is dependent on the strength of the horse's immune system, the dose of the bacteria, and the strain of the bacteria. If it is a complicated case, a mortality rate of up to forty percent is seen (Spaulding, 2010).

PREVENTION

The course of this infection allows for bacterial shedding to occur before abscesses appear, and perhaps even before the onset of fever. This means that this infection can be widely distributed by the time symptoms are observed. Susceptibility to strangles depends on exposure, the host's immune status, and the virulence of the bacterial strain. Risks for exposure to strangles include a large population size that may lead to overcrowding, frequent travel, severe weather, interaction with horses from different areas, concurrent illness, and improper nutrition (Morris Animal Foundation, 2022).

The best strategy to prevent strangles is to minimize exposure risks. Horses that are newly introduced onto a farm should be observed and temperature monitored twice a day for at least two weeks before being housed with resident horses. Horses with temperatures over 101.5 degrees Fahrenheit should be isolated (KBHH, n.d.).

A good way to herbally prevent strangles is to increase the horse's immune system with herbs such as three tablespoons powdered astragalus per day, five teaspoons of garlic per day (about five cloves), two tablespoons powdered turmeric per day, one teaspoon powdered ginseng per day, six to twelve teaspoons goldenseal tincture daily, and one tablespoon powdered echinacea three times a day (Brookby Herbs, 2018).

TREATMENT

In most cases, strangles is treated with rest and supportive care. Horses are monitored closely to ensure adequate consumption of food and water. Feeding wet, sloppy food from the floor also makes it easier for infected horses to swallow and encourages the abscesses to drain (Young, 2020).

Horses that develop lymph node abscesses or have severe cases may require flushing of the abscesses with a diluted apple cider vinegar solution and a second time with a calendula herbal tea once the abscesses have opened. Hot compressing of the abscesses will also help to bring them to the surface, allowing them to rupture (Young 2020).

Affected horses should be quarantined and all movement of horses on and off the property halted until all horses that had contact with the infected horse are confirmed to be negative (Young, 2020).

Nasal shedding of the bacteria can persist for up to three weeks and horses may be infectious for at least six weeks after nasal discharge has stopped (Spaulding, 2010).

Comfrey leaves may help with strangles because of its wonderful effects on the respiratory system. Give forty leaves per day for an average 1100-pound horse (Young, 2020).

If the horse has a strong immune system and a good clean environment, strangles is not commonly seen. See above in the prevention section to understand good herbs to boost the horse's immune system and also the immune system in chapter 6.

TETANUS (Lockjaw)

Tetanus, or lockjaw, is a frequently fatal non-contagious neurological disease that results from a bacterial infection. The bacterial spores can be found everywhere in the environment and can survive long periods, making it particularly dangerous for horses (Spaulding, 2010).

Unfortunately, horses are more sensitive to tetanus infection than with other animals including cattle, dogs, and humans. Tetanus can survive in a horse undetected for long periods without causing infection or clinical signs (Spaulding, 2010).

These spores enter the horse's body through a skin wound or through ulcers in the gastrointestinal tract after ingesting infected feces. It may take anywhere between seven and thirty days to show symptoms in a horse (Spaulding, 2010).

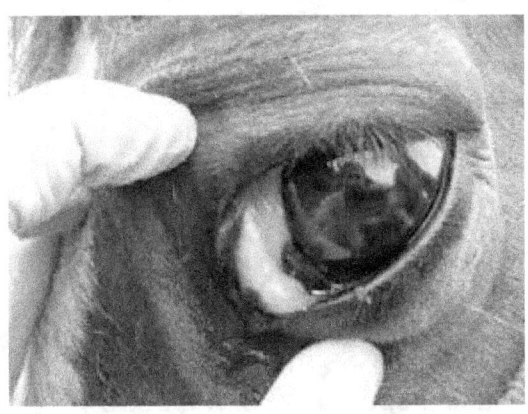

It can cause general stiffness, muscle spasms, difficulty chewing, difficulty swallowing, difficulty drinking, third eyelid prolapse (protrusion of pink tissue from the corner of the eye), sensitive to touch, sweating, fever, convulsions, 'sawhorse' stance, respiratory arrest, and death (Spaulding, 2010).

The prognosis for affected horses is generally very poor with only a twenty percent survival rate. An underweight horse may struggle even more. Horses that survive and stand for the first seven to ten days of the disease have a better prognosis (Spaulding, 2010).

PREVENTION

Maintaining a healthy gastrointestinal tract and preventing ulcers may help ward off tetanus infection by limiting entry sites into the circulatory system (McNeil, 2023).

Keeping hooves clean and away from injury may be another way to help ward off tetanus as a small cut or abrasion can allow the Tetanus bacteria into the horse's system (Young, 2020).

Always ensure that paddocks, stalls and pastures are free of debris and materials that could potentially cause an injury. This includes but is not limited to rusty metal, old farm equipment and sharp edges on fences, feeders and waterers (Spaulding, 2010).

TREATMENT

Loud sounds, bright lights, excitement in their surroundings and touch can make symptoms worse and overstimulate affected horses. The horse should be kept in a quiet, dark stall. This may help prevent anxiety and reduce muscle spasms (Young, 2020).

Horses with tetanus are often stiff and unable to bend down. All food and water sources in the stall should be kept at a height that allows use without having to move the head up or down (Young, 2020).

In modern medicine, there is a Tetanus vaccine that can be administered. Of course, any type of vaccine will decrease the horse's immune system and make the liver work harder to metabolize the chemical toxin introduced into their system (Young, 2020).

Even with herbal treatment, this is a major situation the horse goes through. Getting herbs into their system to increase the immune system and to act as an antibiotic is a must. These herbs include three tablespoons powdered astragalus per day, five teaspoons of garlic per day (about five cloves), two tablespoons powdered turmeric per day, one teaspoon of powdered ginseng per day, six to twelve teaspoons of goldenseal tincture daily, and one tablespoon powdered echinacea three times a day (Young, 2020). (See chapter 6: Immune System)

In addition to these herbs, adding herbs that will help with muscle contractions may also help. A really great herb to help with muscle spasms and strain is called cramp bark. Cramp bark is best made into a tincture and then drenched for a horse (three teaspoons every four to six hours). Adult horses should be given two powdered tablespoons three or four times a day (Homegrown Herbalist, n.d.).

ARTHRITIS/DEGENERATIVE JOINT DISEASE

Arthritis is unfortunately very common in horses, especially in the ageing horse population. It is a degenerative joint disease that causes pain and inflammation. Over time, the inflammation damages the cartilage within a joint beyond repair, leading to chronic pain (Horse Health Programe, 2023).

Cartilage is the 'cushioning' within a joint which allows it to run smoothly. Arthritis is unfortunately not curable and instead must be managed for the rest of a horse's life (Scone Equine Hospital, n.d.).

Arthritis is one of the most common causes of retirement amongst horses, so early diagnosis and management is really important. Most commonly, a horse will show signs of swelling or heat around the affected joint, lameness, pain on joint flexion, subtle changes to their actions, wider limb stance, changing of lead legs, reluctance to work, or mild stiffness initially that may improve with exercise (Horse Health Programe, 2023).

PREVENTION

Prevention is solely based on what has caused the arthritis. Managing the horse's weight is one way to help prevent arthritis. Overweight horses carry extra pounds around which adds stress and strain to their joints (Scone Equine Hospital, n.d.).

Exercise is also very important. If arthritic joints are seen, a regular routine of gentle exercise may benefit them. When a horse stands in their stable for extended periods of time without exercise, it can cause the horse's joints to become increasingly stiff and sore and cause arthritic degeneration to begin (Scone Equine Hospital, n.d.).

TREATMENT

Yucca is one of the popular herbs that many horse owners consider for arthritis and joint support. It contains saponins, which are natural compounds known for their anti-inflammatory properties. One to two tablespoons of powdered yucca can be mixed into their feed daily to help with arthritic joints (Kaufman's, n.d.).

Another plant that contains beneficial elements for joint health is turmeric. It has an active compound called curcumin which has potent anti-inflammatory and antioxidant benefits. Two to three powdered teaspoons into their feed should be sufficient (Stronach, 2023).

Devil's Claw is also used for its anti-inflammatory effects. A dosage of one powdered teaspoon twice a day is recommended (Horse Health Programe, 2023).

Boswellia is yet another herb with anti-inflammatory properties and is praised for its potential to improve mobility in horses with arthritis. Like yucca and turmeric, a half to one teaspoon of powdered boswellia can be added directly to the feed your horse already consumes (Reverdy, n.d.).

Comfrey is known to have healing effects with arthritis. Providing this internally and externally is the best route. Forty leaves a day is a good dosage for a horse. Topically, you can use a comfrey tincture spray, comfrey poultice, herbal infused oil, or herbal salve (Homegrown Herbalist, n.d.).

LAMANITIS

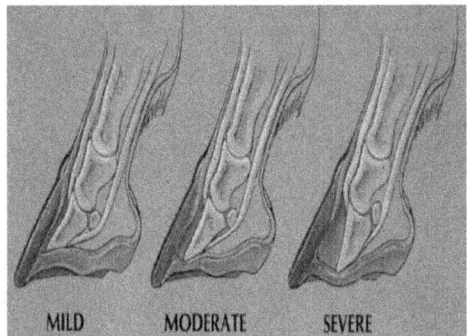

MILD   MODERATE   SEVERE

Laminitis is damage and inflammation of the tissue between the hoof and the underlying bone. This tissue, the laminae (also called lamellae), is actually folded layers of tissue, contacting the surface of the bone on one side and the inside of the hoof wall on the other, connecting the two (Horse Herbs, n.d.).

Depending on how severely these attachments are weakened, the outcome can range from mild foot soreness to separation of the bone and hoof. The front hooves, which bear the majority of the horse's weight, are most commonly affected, but it can also occur in the hind hooves (Horse Herbs, n.d.).

Laminitis can be the outcome of excessive grain intake, access to pasture high in sugars, compensatory weight bearing due to injury of the opposite limb, ingestion of toxic plants (such as black walnut), and excessive work on hard surfaces such as pavement (Horse Herbs, n.d.).

The clinical signs of laminitis vary depending on the amount of damage to the laminae. Lameness with variable severity in one or more hooves is common. Affected horses may be reluctant to move or unwilling to rise. When standing, they may shift their weight from one hoof to another, or stand with their front feet out in front of them and hind feet under their bodies ("sawhorse stance") (Horse Herbs, n.d.).

PREVENTION

Prevention includes limiting access to lush pastures which can be high in sugars, minimizing sugar and carbohydrates in their diet, maintaining proper hoof care, providing limb support for the opposite leg if one is injured, and keeping the horses weight at a healthy limit (Young, 2020).

TREATMENT

Laminitis is irreversible and once clinical signs are observed, the damage is already underway. At this point, it is important to minimize further progression (Young, 2020).

Horses may be placed on stall rest with deep bedding in severe cases. Cold therapy in the form of ice baths or boots may also be utilized to minimize inflammation (Horse Herbs, n.d.).

Herbs that are great for laminitis relief in an 1100-pound horse are two tablespoons powdered nettle leaf daily, one tablespoon powdered hawthorn leaf daily (Horse Herbs, n.d.), two tablespoons fenugreek seeds daily, two tablespoons powdered yarrow daily, two to three tablespoons rosehips daily, two powdered tablespoons cleavers daily (Horse Herbs, n.d.), and forty leaves of comfrey per day (Homegrown Herbalist, n.d.).

BACK PROBLEMS

Back problems are a major cause of poor performance and gait abnormalities. There are all types of problems that can happen with horses. These include fractures, strains, sprains, ligament pulls, kissing spine syndrome, degenerative spine diseases, or sacroiliac injuries. They can occur from injury or lack of proper vitamins and minerals in their diet (Akers, 2023).

Symptoms include poor performance/reduced performance which may progress to behavioral problems (rearing/bucking/stopping or running out at fences). Many horses will feel "disconnected" from front to back, or may have a short strided gait in general (Clegg, 2022).

Discomfort to grooming or pressure over the back or when saddling are other symptoms. This should be interpreted with caution because some horses may simply be "thin skinned" and may not be experiencing significant back pain. However, a sudden change in your horse's response to grooming may be an indicator of back pain (University of Minnesota Extension, 2023).

PREVENTION
Sometimes horses are born with abnormalities and there is not a way to prevent this from happening (Clegg, 2022).

Deficiency in proper vitamins and minerals is one-way horses can develop degenerative back issues. Making sure they have the correct type and amount of feed, water, and grazing pasture is crucial (Clegg, 2022).

The amount of weight saddled and how overweight a horse or their owner are, are things that play apart in preventing back problems. Don't saddle more weight than the horse can handle and also keep check of the horse's weight (University of Minnesota Extension, 2023).

Stretching is also a good way to prevent back problems. If a horse is exercised regularly, they have less chance of muscle atrophy or other clinical problems that could result in back problems (University of Minnesota Extension, 2023).

TREATMENT
The best way to treat a back problem is to first know what is causing the pain your horse is experiencing and then treat with herbal pain relievers (Finish Line Horse Products, 2018). Two great herbal pain relievers are white willow bark and Devil's Claw. Two tablespoons powdered white willow bark daily and one teaspoon of powdered devil's claw two times daily is recommended (The Horse Herbalist, 2016).

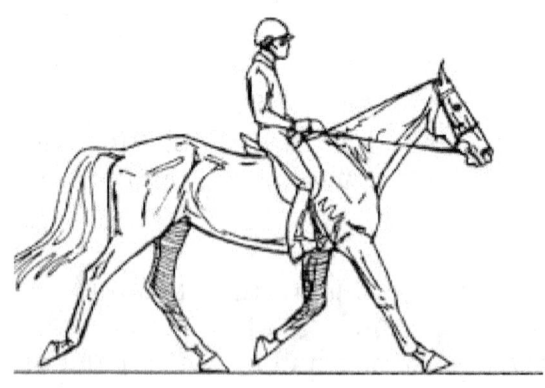

DEGENERATIVE SUSPENSORY LIGAMENT
(Desmitis)

Desmitis is a genetically inherited chronic condition in horses that affects connective tissue, ligaments, and tendons. This painful condition commonly leads to debilitating lameness. It is caused by not having the specific proteins and collagen fibers in their system to repair ligaments (Conley Koontz Equine Hospital, n.d.).

Signs of desmitis include tripping and stumbling, constant stomping not caused by flies, frequently lying down, instability that may appear neurologic in nature, back soreness as the horse changes stance to relieve limb pain, sitting on fences or other objects to obtain pain relief, shifting back and forth to gain relief, irritability, digging a hole in the pasture and stands with the toes pointing towards the hole, assuming a dog position before getting up from laying down, having loose skin, having white hair spots, and other behavioral changes (Meggitt, 2023).

PREVENTION

Because desmitis is a genetic disorder, there is no way of preventing this from occurring, although horses with this disease should not be bred (Darani, 2020).

TREATMENT

Unfortunately, there is currently no cure and there are no reliable measures to slow disease progression. Supportive care includes corrective shoeing, controlled exercise plans, no prolonged stall rest, and a well-balanced diet, including proper vitamin and mineral intake (Darani, 2020).

An herb that has been shown to greatly help with pain associated with desmitis is called Jiaogulan. Jiaogulan is a climbing vine that helps a horse with circulation, vitality, gait, hoof health, respiratory health, and muscle function. The typical dosage is one powdered teaspoon twice daily. This herb should be introduced slowly to minimize avoidance (Darani, 2020).

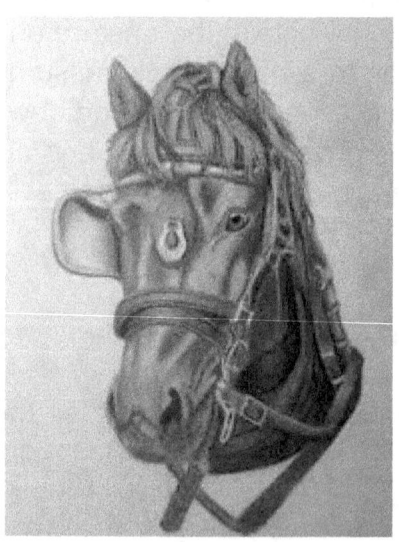

PITUITARY PARS INTERMEDIA DYSFUNCTION
(PPID) (Cushing's Disease)

Equine Cushing's disease involves the pituitary gland, which is a gland located at the base of the brain that produces hormones in response to brain signals. It affects those over the age of ten, with nineteen being the average age at diagnosis (Afzul, 2021).

In PPID, the normal mechanisms which control hormone production by the pituitary gland are damaged causing excessive production of the normal hormones from the pituitary. These hormones then enter the circulation and affect the whole body (Afzul, 2021).

Signs of this disease include increased coat length and delayed shedding of the winter coat, laminitis, lethargy, increased sweating, weight loss, and excessive drinking and urinating (Afzul, 2021).

PREVENTION

Prevention includes giving your horse a balanced diet and exercise. Observe hair growth and keep an eye on your horse's coat. An abnormal, persistent winter coat could be an early indicator of the disease (Afzal, 2021).

TREATMENT

One herb that is great for Cushing's in horses is two and a half teaspoons Chaste tree berries daily. It's believed that the herb stimulates production of the chemical mediator dopamine, which regulates production of the pituitary gland (Herbs for horses, 2023).

Dopamine producing cells in normal horses are limited in their antioxidation capacity in horses with Cushing's and therefore herbs that are natural in anti-oxidants are really great. Some of those include two to three teaspoons rosehips per day (Rose-Hip Vital, n.d.), two tablespoons powdered turmeric per day, one fourth cup powdered green tea per day, two teaspoons grape seed oil extract, and three tablespoons powdered hawthorn daily are also rich sources of natural anti-oxidants (Honeyvale Herbs, n.d.).

Because organs are put under extreme pressure by the disease, one tablespoon powdered cayenne daily and four tablespoons powdered nettle daily are extremely beneficial for circulation. One teaspoon milk thistle seeds for two-three times a day and two cups powdered dandelion leaves daily are wonderful for the liver and kidneys (ESC, n.d.). One teaspoon of bilberries daily and one teaspoon powdered eyebright daily are also recommended to improve eyesight (Honeyvale Herbs, n.d.).

Horses with Cushing's disease can become deficient in many minerals and amino acids because they urinate frequently. It is always a good idea to add one tablespoon kelp in their diet per day to support their endocrine system (Stronach, 2023). They also have an increased risk of infection because of elevated blood sugar levels. For this, five teaspoons' garlic (about five cloves) and three powdered tablespoons calendula are recommended (Royal Veterinary College, n.d.).

FOAL PNEUMONIA

Rhodococcus equi, a naturally occurring bacterium in soil, is the most devastating cause of pneumonia in foals up to six months of age. It affects the lungs and airways, causing disturbances in respiration and deficiency of oxygen in the blood (Rush, 2022).

Signs include lethargy, fever, and rapid breathing. Cough is an occasional sign, while pus-containing nasal discharge is less common. Sometimes crackles and wheezes in the chest can be heard. Some foals will have inflamed joints as well (Holistachorse, n.d.).

PREVENTION

Foals should be maintained in a well-ventilated and dust-free area with avoidance to dirt paddocks and overcrowding. Foals with pneumonia should be isolated and their manure composted (Rush, 2022).

TREATMENT

Mullein is a great herb for irritated and inflamed airways. One tablespoon daily of finely powdered mullein is adequate for a foal up to five hundred pounds. Make sure to finely powder the mullein leaves because the fuzzy covering of the leaves can actually be irritating to the horse's mouth and lips (Rush, 2022).

Peppermint can help with breathing and the immune system. It also has a calming and cooling action to settle horses that are agitated and restless. Add two teaspoons powdered peppermint into their feed daily (Feed XL Equine Nutrition Team, n.d.).

Rosehips, marshmallow root, comfrey leaves, and fenugreek seeds all help with infections of the respiratory systems (Great Southern Stock Feeds, n.d.). One tablespoon rosehips daily (Rose-Hip Vital, n.d.), two teaspoons powdered marshmallow root (Horse Meds, n.d.), twenty leaves of fresh comfrey leaves, and two teaspoons fenugreek seeds can be given to a foal daily to help with their lungs (Foxden Equine, 2023).

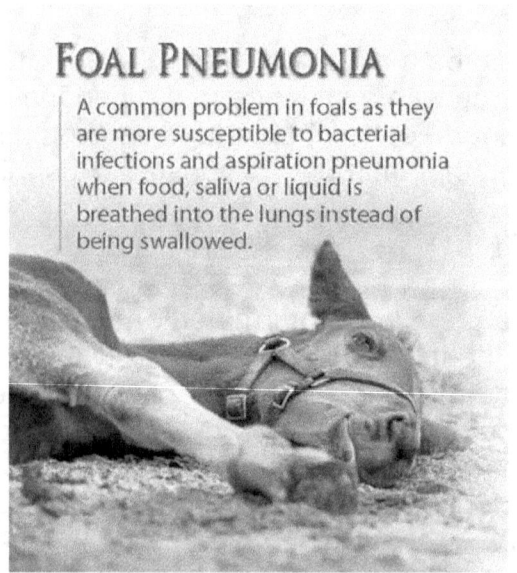

FOAL PNEUMONIA
A common problem in foals as they are more susceptible to bacterial infections and aspiration pneumonia when food, saliva or liquid is breathed into the lungs instead of being swallowed.

POTOMAC HORSE FEVER

Potomac horse fever (PHF) is caused by the Neorickettsia risticii bacteria (formerly known as Ehrlichia risticii). Potomac horse fever can cause diarrhea, gastrointestinal upsets, abortions in pregnant mares, and sometimes death (Chahan, 2023).

The horse gets the bacteria when drinking from creeks, rivers or ponds in the summer months that is laced with a particular bacterium. Other common signs are depression, anorexia, and fever (Chahan, 2023).

PREVENTION

Providing clean drinking water, eliminating standing water sources where insects may breed, and turning off stable lighting at night that may attract insects can all help prevent Potomac horse fever (Lenher, n.d.).

TREATMENT

Giloy herb helps to prevent infections and eliminates the causative agents from the horse's body. Two powdered tablespoons can be given two times a day (Lenher, n.d.).

Ashwagandha is another good herb to give strength to the horse's body and helps he/she fight any weakness. Two powdered tablespoons can be given two times a day (Lenher, n.d.).

SALMONELLA

Salmonella is one of the most common bacterial diseases of adult horses. Infection can occur via contamination of the environment, feed or water, or by contact with animals actively shedding the bacteria. Infected animals also can be asymptomatic and continue to shed the bacteria intermittently. The most common signs include fever, lethargy, diarrhea, anorexia, and colic (University of Minnesota Extension, n.d.).

PREVENTION

Keep horses away from areas where other horses may be such as horse shows and other events. As the horse's owner, wash your hands frequently and don't share equipment between horses (Young, 2020).

TREATMENT

Garlic is widely used in horses as an antibiotic, although large doses can be toxic. Five teaspoons of garlic or equivalent to five small cloves, can be given to a horse daily along with one forth cup powdered chamomile twice a day. Chamomile acts as an antispasmodic to assist in soothing inflammation (Natural Solutions, 2023).

MANGE

Mange is caused by microscopic mites that invade the skin of horses. The mites cause irritation of the skin and a hypersensitivity reaction, resulting in itching, hair loss, and inflammation. While there are several different types of mange that affect horses, it is rare (Spaulding, 2010).

One of the most common types of mange is leg mange. It tends to occur in heavy (draft) breeds. Signs begin as itching around the hind legs and foot. Raised bumps, hair loss, crusting, and thickening of the skin can be seen, however the actual mites that cause mange can't be seen by the naked human eye (Spaulding, 2010).

PREVENTION

Birds can carry certain species on their wing when they visit stables and can infect a horse. A good way to prevent the birds from visiting your horse is to plant herbs that will deter birds. Those deterring herbs and other plants are garlic, onions, thorny plants, citronella, mint, basil, sage, rosemary, marjoram, lavender, pennyroyal, thyme, and daffodils DeAngelis, 2022).

Horses can also get mange from other infected horses or infected humans. Making sure to keep horses separated and using good hygiene is always a plus when working with horses (Horton, 2019).

TREATMENT

Feeding your horse garlic can help deter a lot of pests. Feed your horse five teaspoons or five small cloves of garlic a day. You can also crush the liquid from the garlic to dab on your horse as a topical repellant. Also try some powdered comfrey leaf mixed with a dab of water topically to make a poultice or you can topically use a spray comfrey leaf tincture (WorldHorseWelfare, n.d.).

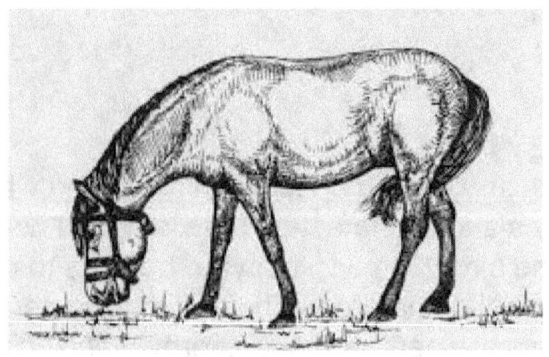

THRUSH

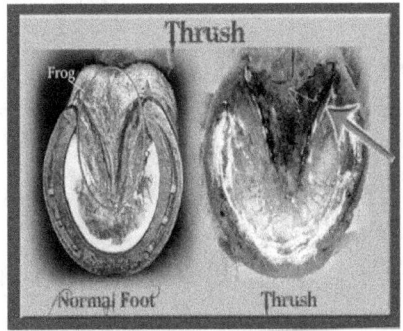

Thrush is a common bacterial infection of the horse's hoof tissue characterized by a black, necrotic (dead), foul-smelling material. It can be caused by abnormal hoof growth, lack of trimming or shoeing, lack of movement, and poor circulation in the hoof (Spaulding, 2010).

Classic signs of thrush include a thick, black, puttylike material on or in the hoof. Limping may also be observed (Spaulding, 2010).

PREVENTION

Although thrush can't always be prevented if the hoof has grown abnormally or with already known circulation problems. In a normal horse hoof, making sure to trim the hooves periodically is imperative. It is also imperative that the horse has plenty of exercise to work the hooves (Arizona Equine, 2016).

TREATMENT

Cleaning the affected foot and/or feet daily is a must. You must make sure it is as dry as possible before applying herbal medication. The foot can, on occasion, be scrubbed gently with water and a stiff brush (Spaulding, 2010).

Herbal medication includes making an oil with the tea tree. Applying this topically can help increase the immune system while decreasing inflammation. Comfrey leaves can also be used topically if powdered and made into a paste or sprayed on as a topical tincture (Arizona Equine, 2016).

~~~~~~

MUD FEVER

Mud fever, also known as pastern dermatitis or 'cracked heels' is characterized by scabs and sores on a horse's legs. It often affects pink skinned areas and may be noticed as red, sore areas of skin that may be weeping, or lumpy patches often on the lower limbs, although any leg can be affected (Scott Dunn's Equine Clinic, n.d.).

Left untreated, mud fever can develop into costly complications if an infection travels up the leg through the damaged skin, causing a painful condition known as cellulitis (Scott Dunn's Equine Clinic, n.d.).

This painful skin condition is caused by bacteria that live in the environment. Wet, damaged skin provides an ideal moist environment for the bacteria to grow (Scott Dunn's Equine Clinic, n.d.).

Once an infection develops, this can cause the skin to be very itchy and the horse may scratch their legs, damaging the skin's protective barrier further and promoting penetration of more bacteria into the skin.

Horses with hairy feathered legs are typically at risk as the hair will trap moisture against the skin (Scott Dunn's Equine Clinic, n.d.).

PREVENTION

Avoiding wet, muddy conditions will help prevent mud fever. This includes gateways, shelters, and pastures. You can better achieve this by placing woodchips onto these muddy conditions (Scott Dunn's Equine Clinic, n.d.).

Clipping of hairy legs can be very useful as it facilitates keeping the legs clean and dry, and provides better visibility so any lesions are likely to be noticed and treated earlier (Scott Dunn's Equine Clinic, n.d.).

Keeping legs clean and dry is imperative. Wet skin provides the perfect conditions for the bacteria to grow and multiply (Scott Dunn's Equine Clinic, n.d.).

TREATMENT

Arnica is an herb that can help with wounds. Make a salve and apply it topically daily. Also, the use of tea tree oil topically can also help decrease the inflammation. Internally, it is recommended to use five cloves of garlic or five small cloves daily and two tablespoons of white willow bark daily (Mane Event, n.d.).

WOUNDS/CUTS

Wounds and/or cuts in horses are unfortunately extremely common. The most common wounds occur on horse's limbs and are caused by foreign objects such as fences, gates, farm equipment, and building materials. Wounds on the distal (lower) limbs of horses can be especially difficult to manage because of poor circulation, joint movement and minimal soft tissue between skin and bone (Rossdales Veterinary Surgeons, n.d.).

Wounds on the distal (lower) limbs of horses can be especially difficult to manage because of poor circulation, joint movement and minimal soft tissue between skin and bone. There is also always the risk of contamination from the environment. The smallest most innocuous looking cut or puncture wound can sometimes present a serious problem (Rossdales Veterinary Surgeons, n.d.).

There are three main types of wounds: Puncture wounds, lacerations, and abrasions. Abrasions are generally minor wounds that require cleaning and can be treated topically. Lacerations may cause underlying soft tissue damage and infection. Puncture wounds may look small on the surface, but there may be significant damage beneath the skin surface. These may be complicated by infection, as contamination is introduced deep into the wound. Often, the skin heals before the underlying tissue (Rossdales Veterinary Surgeons, n.d.).

PREVENTION

Because horse wounds occur mostly from fences, gates, farm equipment, and building supplies, it is important for you to make sure such things are out of the horses reach and in good repair (Horse, Herbs, n.d.).

TREATMENT

With any type of wound, wash it thoroughly with cold water. This will also help reduce any swelling. If the horse is bleeding, use a compaction of the herb called yarrow. Yarrow flowers will stop bleeding (Horse Herbs, n.d.).

If you can do it safely without further injuring the horse, or yourself, clip the hair around the wound. This will help to assess the wound and keep it clean (Horse Herbs, n.d.).

The most effective healing herb for a surface wound is comfrey. This is an amazing herb because of the allantoin found in the roots and leaves. Allantoin is a substance that reduces inflammation, helps new skin cells grow, and keeps the skin healthy. Comfrey can be given to a horse internally or topically. If using internally, about forty leaves will help clear any infection inside the horse and topically, it will help heal the wound very quickly (Horse Herbs, n.d.).

Because comfrey works so well and so quickly at healing, it should never be used on a puncture wound. A puncture wound is very deep and therefore the surface of the skin will heal before the inside layers has a chance to heal. This will cause infection and a lot of issues (Spaulding, 2010).

Manuka honey is also great for wounds. Any honey will work, however specifically manuka honey has healing qualities that can't be beat. Topical use helps to fight infections and speeds recovery (Schell, n.d.).

Calendula is great for horse's skin. It is primarily recognized for its antiseptic, detoxification, and healing properties. It helps prevent the spread of infection, quickens recovery time, combats fevers, and fights infections (Mane Event, n.d.).

With any wounds or cuts, it is a good idea to use calendula flowers topically and internally. Most horses will find calendula flowers highly palatable. Dried calendula may be added directly to your horse's feed or be made into a tea. The tea can be poured over their feed or into their water bucket (Horse Herbs, n.d.).

One other one to mention is cayenne pepper. While cayenne pepper may have a 'kick' at the beginning, using it topically on a horses wound can help relieve the pain. When applying, only add a small amount. It will burn for a few seconds so be mindful the horse may kick and try to get away from it. Once it soaks in, the horse will find relief (Horse Herbs, n.d.).

Applying a salve or poultice topically of either the comfrey, calendula, manuka honey, or powdered cayenne pepper can be challenging. Depending on where the wound is located on the horse's body, a dressing can be applied with the salve and/or poultice underneath (Spaulding, 2010).

Ideally the dressing should be applied with firm pressure, but not too tight to restrict blood flow. If it is too loose, it may not stay in place. The dressing should be changed frequently to reduce inflammation and possible infection (Horse Herbs, n.d.).

BITES/STINGS

Bites and stings on a horse is almost a given. Anything from flies, mosquitos, bees, wasps, spider, etc. will most likely happen. Signs include scratching, biting, and rubbing of the skin, sometimes with loss of hair on the body, mane and tail. Some horses may be so severely affected that they may have weight loss or show behavioral changes such as restlessness and irritability (Wishgarden, 2018).

PREVENTION

To help prevent bites and stings from occuring, it is a good idea to have frequent manure removal, eliminating standing water, and bringing your horse inside during peak insect feeding times. Large, strong box fans can also help prevent bites from insect species that are weak fliers (Wishgarden, 2018).

TREATMENT

There are five herbs that stand out for a bite or sting with a horse. The first one is peppermint. Peppermint oil or crushed leaves are cooling and can soothe itchy or inflamed bites. Simply place a peppermint herbal oil onto the sting or bite and allow it to penetrate the area or make a poultice with the crushed leaves and apply a dressing. Change the dressing often (Wishgarden, 2018).

Calendula flower oil or fresh leaves can soothe irritated, itchy skin, and can encourage healthy healing of bites and stings. A simple salve can be created with calendula and beeswax and applied to the wound (Pro Equine Grooms, n.d.).

Witch hazel is an herb that can help relieve minor skin irritations. Create an itch-soothing poultice and apply topically with a dressing that you change frequently. Be careful with witch hazel as the horse should not eat it. Make sure the horse can't reach the dressing with their mouth (Pro Equine Grooms, n.d.).

Comfrey infused oil or fresh juice from leaves can be used topically for bites and stings on a horse. It helps to soothe itching and irritation. Simply apply with a poultice, spray on tincture, or salve (Pro Equine Grooms, n.d.).

And last, but certainly not least, there is plantain. Not to be confuse with the banana leaf, plantain herb is an amazing herb for pulling out the toxins from bee stings or snake bites. It grows almost anywhere and many refer to it as an obnoxious weed. It has a powerful anti-bacterial effect and contains allantoin which is a phytochemical that speeds up wound healing and stimulates the growth of new skin cells. It also helps to stop bleeding, sooth pain, and relieve itching (Pro Equine Grooms, n.d.).

Plantain works best if you can apply a generous amount as soon as the bite or sting happens. It is always best to have a spray-on tincture ready for use, however simply picking the plantain leaves, crushing them in your mouth (mixed with your salvia) can make a spit poultice perfect in a situation where you need to quickly apply a poultice to draw out the poison (Pro Equine Grooms, n.d.).

PARASITES (WORMS)

Internal parasites (worms) are organisms that live in pastures and also internally inside a horse and ingest the horses' nutrients. The horse is affected by many different species of parasites (Spaulding, 2010).

A horse can be quite severely infested with worms and have few or no symptoms visible to the naked eye (Spaulding, 2010). It's a good idea to regularly test the horse's manure to know if they have worms and what type of worms they have in their system (College of Veterinary Medicine, 2018). You can do this by sending a fecal sample to your veterinarian but you can also educate yourself with what the worms look like and purchase a microscope to determine worm load count (Spaulding, 2010).

If pharmaceutical medication is used to deworm frequently, some worms can develop a resistance. If you go that route, don't deworm until fecal analysis shows the types of worms you should be deworming (Spaulding, 2010).

The primary class of internal parasites that cause health problems for horses are nematodes (such as large and small strongyles), roundworms and tapeworms. Other internal parasites of minor significance include threadworms, pinworms and botfly larvae (Lombardi, 2021).

Signs of parasites include weight loss, dull, rough hair coat, potbelly, decreased stamina, lethargy, coughing, diarrhea, colic, and tail rubbing (Hiney, 2017).

Pinworms especially causes the horse to rub their hind end on water buckets, feeders, and other objects because they itch when they exit the horse's body to lay eggs (College of Veterinary Medicine, 2018).

PREVENTION

Regular rotation of pastures in one way to help prevent parasites. This will help lower the worm burden, as well as give forage a chance to recover. Grouping horses in pastures according to age will also help minimize young horses' exposure to ascarids (roundworms) and other parasites. If possible, pasture cattle, sheep or goats behind the horse(s). These species will consume the infective larvae of the horses' parasites (Hiney, 2017). One other way to help prevent parasites is harrowing your pastures. This 'dragging' is only recommended during extremely hot, dry conditions and when horses can be removed from the pasture for a minimum of two weeks (Giedt, E., 2017).

Make sure the horses stall in cleaned on a regular basis and the manure in composted (Giedt, E., 2017). Food grade diatomaceous earth may be a good option to sprinkle around the horse stalls. Diatomaceous earth is made from the fossilized remains of tiny, aquatic organisms called diatoms. Their skeletons are made of a natural substance called silica. Over a long period of time, diatoms accumulated in the sediment of rivers, streams, lakes, and oceans (Npic, n.d.).

TREATMENT

Natural dewormers are either vermicides or vermifuges. Vermicides kill the parasite whereas vermifuges numbs the parasite so that it can easily be flushed from the body (Lombardi, 2021). Some really great vermicides and vermifuges that should be given no more than one week and then reevaluated are one tablespoon of dried and crushed fennel seeds daily, thirty-six crushed cloves twice a day, four tablespoons ground echinacea daily (Brookby Herbs, 2018), six tablespoons of cayenne pepper twice a day for three days (then to six tablespoons once a week for prevention), no more than twenty-five percent of their diet of red clover (Giedt, 2017), four cloves of garlic per day, one cup crushed ginger root daily, six to eight drops of oregano oil mixed into water daily and drenched, four tablespoons crushed rosemary daily, fifteen grams powdered sage per day, four tablespoons crushed thyme daily, two cups squash seeds daily, and two cups pumpkin seeds daily (Verm Oust, 2019).

If you have enjoyed this book, this information, along with nine other animals, will be available in "Herbal Animal Care for the Homesteader" which will be available on Amazon, Books-A-Million, Barnes and Noble, and many other popular bookstores soon. I appreciate the purchase of this book. I wish nothing but the best health for your horse!

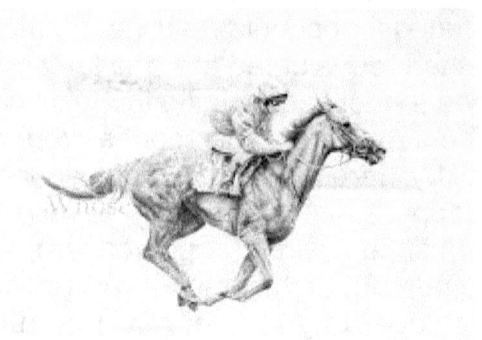

References

Afzal, S. (2021, October 25). *Equine Cushing's Care Guide: From Early Signs to Holistic Management*. Poll to Pasture Holistics. https://www.polltopastern.com/post/equine-cushing-s-disease#:~:text=Preventative%20Care%3A%20Implement%20preventative%20care,early%20indicator%20of%20the%20disease.

Akers, C. (n.d.). *Standard Process - Equine Metabolic Syndrome Supplements*. https://journeysholisticlife.com/blogs/resources/standard-process-equine-metabolic

Apfel, K. (2018, May 8). *10 Amazing Facts...About Insect Repelling Plants*. https://horse-canada.com/magazine/farm-management/10-insect-repelling-plants/

Apelian, N. (2021). *The Lost Book of Herbal Remedies*. pp. 33-42

Argyle Veterinary Hospital (n.d.). *Equine Influenza: Symptoms and Treatment of the Flu in Horses*. https://www.argylevet.com/site/blog/2021/09/22/equine-influenza#:~:text=Treatment%20for%20equine%20influenza%20involves,respiratory%20tract%20to%20adequately%20heal

Arizona Equine (2016, April 15). *What is Thrush in Horses?* https://azequine.com/thrush/#:~:text=Thrush%20is%20a%20common%20anaerobic,)%2C%20foul%2Dsmelling%20material.

Britannica. (n.d.). *Black Walnut*. https://www.britannica.com/plant/black-walnut

Brookby Herbs (2018, December 15). *Echinacea: An Aid on Fighting Infections in Horses*. https://brookbyherbs.com/blogs/news/echinacea-an-aid-on-fighting-infections-in-horses

Brookby Herbs (2018, April 21). *Horse Colic Treatment - Peppermint may be part of the answer*. https://brookbyherbs.com/blogs/news/horse-colic-treatment-peppermint-may-be-part-of-the-answer#:~:text=Because%20Peppermint%20is%20anti%2Dinflammatory,enjoy%20the%20sweet%20aroma%20yourself.

Brookby Herbs (2018, September 27). *Strangles in Horses – What To Do*. https://brookbyherbs.com/blogs/news/strangles-in-horses-what-to-do

Chahan, V. (2022, March 3). *What is Potomac Horse Fever?- Diagnosis, Symptoms and Herbal Supplements*. https://www.planetayurveda.net/herbal-supplements-for-potomac-horse-fever/

Chahan, V. (2023, June 6). *Equine Influenza in Horses- Causes, Symptoms, and Its Herbal Treatment*. https://www.planetayurveda.net/equine-influenza-in-horses-its-herbal-treatment/

Clegg, P. (2022, October). *Disorders of the Back in Horses*. https://www.merckvetmanual.com/horse-owners/bone,-joint,-and-muscle-disorders-in-horses/disorders-of-the-back-in-horses

Coates, J. (2012, October 25). *The History and Use of Herbal Medicine and its Use Today with Pets.* https://www.petmd.com/blogs/fullyvetted/2012/oct/history_and_use_of_herbal_medi cine_and_use_in_pets-29279

College of Veterinary Medicine (2018, August 9). *Prevent Parasites, Reduce Problems for your Horse.* https://vetmed.illinois.edu/2018/08/09/horse-worms-parasites/#:~:text=The%20most%20common%20clinical%20sign,%2C%20feeders %2C%20and%20other%20objects.

Conley Koontz Equine Hospital (n.d.) *Degenerative Suspensory Ligament Desmitis (DSLD).* https://www.ckequinehospital.com/page/184/Degenerative-Suspensory-Ligament-Desmitis-DSLD#:~:text=Genetic%20and%20environmental%20factors%20are,systemic%20 proteoglycan%20accumulation%20(ESPA).

Country Park Herbs (n.d.). *Herbal Respiratory Support for All This Smoke.* https://countrypark.com.au/herbal-respiratory-support-with-all-this-smoke/

Crawford, A. (n.d.). *The Flexible Flaxseed.* https://seminolefeed.com/benefits-of-feeding-flaxseed-to-horses/#:~:text=Flaxseed%20is%20generally%20safe%20to,cause%20digestive%2 0upset%20and%20colic.

Darani, P. (2020, November 13). *8 Science-Backed Benefits of Vitamin E in Horses.* https://madbarn.com/vitamin-e-benefits-for-horses/#:~:text=It%20is%20found%20in%20fresh,as%20the%20hay%20is%20stor ed.

Darani, P. (2020). *10 Science-Backed Benefits of Jiaogulan for Horses.* https://madbarn.com/jiaogulan-benefits-for-horses/

DeAngelis, Z. (2022, October 16). *8 Plants That Birds Hate (And How To Use Them).* https://pestpointers.com/plants-that-birds-hate-and-how-to-use-them/

ESC (n.d.). *Dandelion - Depurative and detox action for horses - Pure plant.* https://www.esclaboratoire.com/en/boutique/plantes-pures-chevaux/forme-bien-etre-cheval-plantes/drainage-cheval-plantes/pissenlit-reins-cheval/

Equalite Herbals (2020, March 2). *Echinacea; Boost Your Horse's Immune System and Fight Infection.* https://equiliteherbals.com/blog/echinacea-boost-your-horses-immune-system-and-fight-infection/#:~:text=Boosting%20your%20horse's%20immune%20system,herb%20fo r%20equine%20immune%20support.

Equinews (2013, December 24). *Vitamin C in Horse Diets.* https://ker.com/equinews/vitamin-c-horse-diets/#:~:text=Plants%20are%20a%20natural%20source,as%20they%20begin%20t o%20sprout.

Equus Magazine (2022, March 21). *10 Most Poisonous Plants for Horses.* https://equusmagazine.com/horse-care/10-most-poisonous-plants-for-horses-8208/

Equus Vitalis (n.d.). *Devil's Claw: Good or Bad for Horses?*
https://www.equusvitalis.com/info/magazine/devils-claw-good-or-bad-for-horses#:~:text=How%20much%20Devil's%20Claw%20should,manufacturer%20and%20follow%20them%20closely.

Feed XL Equine Nutrition Team (n.d.). *Herbs: Where do they Fit in Your Horse's Diet?* https://feedxl.com/32-herbs-where-do-they-fit/

Feek, R. (n.d.). *'Why We Homestead', The Homesteading Guide.* pp. 7-11.

Finish Line Horse Products (2018, May 12). *2 Natural Remedies for Managing Horses Pain.* https://finishlinehorse.com/2018/12/2-natural-remedies-for-managing-horses-pain/

Fisher, J. (n.d.). *Osha root: Bear medicine.*
https://www.wintersun.com/blogs/articles/osha-root-bear-medicine

FitAudit (n.d.). *Vitamin E in Spices and Herbs.*
https://fitaudit.com/categories/ssn/vitamin_e

Fox, T. (n.d.). *Goldenseal for Animals – extract.*
https://www.buckmountainbotanicals.net/treatments/goldenseal.html

Foxden Equine (2023, September 19). *Herbal Supplements for Equine Health and Wellness: A Comprehensive Guide to Herbs for Horses.*
https://www.foxdenequine.com/blogs/equine-nutrition/herbal-supplements-for-equine-health-and-wellness-a-comprehensive-guide-to-herbs-for-horses#:~:text=Yucca%20is%20one%20of%20the,for%20their%20anti%2Dinflammatory%20properties.

Funt, R. (n.d.). *Black Walnut Toxicity to Plants, Humans and Horses.*
https://washtenawcd.org/uploads/5/9/2/0/59207889/black_walnut_toxicity_to_plants.pdf

Garland, G. (n.d.). *Equine Respiratory Conditions.*
https://www.wholehorse.com/mullein.html

Giedt, E. (March 2017). *Controlling common internal parasites of the horse.*
https://extension.okstate.edu/fact-sheets/controlling-common-internal-parasites-of-the-horse.html#:~:text=Avoid%20overstocking%20pasture(s)%20as,(roundworms)%20and%20other%20parasites.

Great Southern Stock Feeds, (n.d.). *Rosehip Granules.*
https://greatsouthernstockfeeds.com.au/online-shop/product/182-rosehip-granules#:~:text=In%20Chinese%20herbal%20medicine%20Rosehips,based%20disease%20such%20as%20laminitis.&text=DOSE%3A%202%20tablespoons%20per%20day,size%20and%20level%20of%20work.

Herbs for Horses (2023, November). *Cushing's Care (Pure Chaste Tree Berry).*
https://www.horseherbs.com/products/cushings-care#:~:text=DAILY%20FEED%20RATE%20(per%20500,lbs%20of%20body%20w

eight)%3A&text=Enclosed%20scoop%20is%20approximately%2010g%20(level)%2
0or%2015g%20heaped.

Heeringa, K. (2023, October 25). *Equine Influenza Virus (Flu): Symptoms, Treatment & Prevention.* https://madbarn.com/equine-influenza-virus/#prevention

Hiney, Chris (2017, March). *Common internal parasites of the horse.* https://extension.okstate.edu/fact-sheets/common-internal-parasites-of-the-horse.html

Holistichorse (n.d.). *Herbs to Help Horses Breathe More Easily.* https://holistichorse.com/equine-therapy/herbs-to-help-horses-breathe-more-easily-sp-169132244/

Holistapet (n.d.). *Best Home Remedies for Horse Collic.* https://www.holistapet.com/blogs/horse-care/home-remedies-for-equine-colic

Homegrown Herbalist (n.d.) *Cramp Bark Tincture.* https://homegrownherbalist.net/product/cramp-bark-tincture/

Homesteaddreamer (2017, May 18). *Homestead and Horses: What to Know.* https://www.homesteaddreamer.com/2017/05/18/homesteads-and-horses-what-to-know/#:~:text=Horses%20bring%20a%20variety%20of%20benefits%20to%20homesteads%2C,are%20a%20few%20factors%20to%20think%20about%20beforehand.

Honeyvale Herbs (n.d.). *Herbal Support for Cushing's Disease.* https://honeyvaleherbs.com/herbal-support-cushings-disease/

Honeyvale Herbs (n.d.). *Materia Medica.* https://honeyvaleherbs.com/about-herbs/

Horse Health Programme (n.d.). *Arthritis.* https://www.horsehealthprogramme.co.uk/arthritis/#:~:text=Arthritis%20is%20unfortunately%20very%20common,repair%2C%20leading%20to%20chronic%20pain.

Horse Herbs (n.d.). *Cleaver Herb.* https://www.horseherbs.co.uk/products/cleavers-herb

Horse Herbs (n.d.). *Eyebright.* https://www.horseherbs.co.uk/products/eyebright#:~:text=How%20To%20Feed%20Eyebright,feeds%20or%20given%20at%20once

Horse Herbs (n.d.). *Fenugreek Seeds.* https://www.horseherbs.co.uk/products/fenugreek-powder

Horse Herbs (n.d.). *Hawthorn Leaves.* https://www.horseherbs.co.uk/products/hawthorn-leaves#:~:text=How%20To%20Feed%20Hawthorn%20Leaves,feeds%20or%20given%20at%20once

Horse Herbs (n.d.). *Lami Support Plus.* https://www.horseherbs.co.uk/products/laminitis-relief#:~:text=We%20use%20Cut%20Nettle%20Leaf,is%20added%20or%20taken

%20away.&text=This%20product%20can%20be%20mixed,feeds%20or%20given%20at%20once

Horse Herbs (n.d.). *Marshmallow Root Powder.*
https://www.horseherbs.co.uk/products/marshmallow-root-powder

Horse Herbs (n.d.). *Yarrow Flowers and Leaves (Cut).*
https://www.horseherbs.co.uk/products/yarrow-flowers-leaves-cut#:~:text=How%20To%20Feed%20Yarrow,feeds%20or%20given%20at%20once

The Horse Herbalist (2016, November 26). *Managing the health of the whole horse with herbs.* https://thehorseherbalist.com/managing-the-health-of-the-whole-horse/

Horton, K. (2019, July 18). *Horse Mites 101.*
https://www.equus.co.uk/blogs/community/horse-mites-101#:~:text=How%20do%20horses%20get%20mites,that%20may%20already%20have%20them.

ImmuBiom (2021, January 22). *Equine Immune System.*
https://www.immubiome.com/blogs/horse-resources-and-education/equine-immune-system

Kaufman's (n.d.). *Kaufman's 100% Yucca Powder.* https://ka-hi.com/product/kauffmans-100-yucca-powder-2-lb-pail/#:~:text=Yucca%20powder%20is%20mixed%20with,water%20to%20form%20a%20paste.

KBHH (n.d.). *Strangles Infections are Highly Contagious.* https://www.msd-animal-health-hub.co.uk/Healthy-Horses/Health/AboutStrangles#:~:text=Treatment%20of%20Strangles&text=Feeding%20wet%2C%20sloppy%20food%20from,surface%2C%20allowing%20them%20to%20rupture.

Lenher, E. (n.d.). *Potomac Horse Fever (PHF).*
https://aaep.org/horsehealth/potomac-horse-fever-phf#:~:text=The%20clinical%20manifestations%20of%20PHF,%25%E2%80%9360%25%20of%20cases.

Lentz, Tom (n.d.). *Signs of a Healthy Horse.* https://aaep.org/horsehealth/signs-healthy-horse#:~:text=An%20adult%20horse%20at%20rest,is%2099.5%20%2D%20102.1%20degrees%20Fahrenheit.

Lisa McCann Herbs (n.d.). *Supplier of quality herbs & supplements for horses.*
https://lisamccannherbs.com.au/information/

Lombardi, W. (2021). *Natural Parasite Control For Livestock.* pp.34-53.

Mane Event (n.d.). *Calendula Flowers.*
https://maneeventequestriansupplies.com.au/products/calendula-flowers-1kg#:~:text=Calendula%20Flowers%20(Calendula%20officinalis)%20is,and%20skin%20disorders%20in%20equines.

Mane Event (n.d.). *White Willow Bark Powder.*
https://maneeventequestriansupplies.com.au/products/white-willow-bark-powder-1kg

MacDonald, J. (2018, February 7). *How wild animals self-medicate.*
https://daily.jstor.org/how-wild-animals-self-medicate/

McDowells (n.d.). *Scouring in Horses.*
https://www.mcdowellsherbal.com/treatments/for-horses/701-scouring

McNeil, C. (2023, October 24). *Tetanus in Horses: Signs, Prevention & Treatment.*
https://madbarn.com/tetanus-in-horses/

Meggitt, J. (2023, December 15). *DSLD in Horses [Causes, Management & Prevention].* https://madbarn.com/degenerative-suspensory-ligament-desmitis-in-horses/#:~:text=Degenerative%20Suspensory%20Ligament%20Desmitis%20(DSLD,commonly%20leads%20to%20debilitating%20lameness.

Morris Animal Foundation (2022, December 15). *Bacterial Diseases in Horses.*
https://www.morrisanimalfoundation.org/article/bacteria-infection-disease-horses-foals

Mount Sinai (n.d.). *Comfrey.* https://www.mountsinai.org/health-library/herb/comfrey#:~:text=Comfrey%20(Symphytum%20officinale)%20is%20sometimes,inflammation%20and%20keep%20skin%20healthy.

Mount Sinai (n.d.). *Omega-6 Fatty Acids.* https://www.mountsinai.org/health-library/supplement/omega-6-fatty-acids#:~:text=Along%20with%20omega%2D3%20fatty,and%20maintain%20the%20reproductive%20system.

Natural Solutions (2023, March 10). *Do You Know How Much Garlic To Feed Your Horses?* https://blog.redmondequine.com/do-you-know-how-much-garlic-to-feed-horses#:~:text=So%20how%20much%20garlic%20should,grams%2C%20of%20garlic%20per%20day.

Npic (n.d.) *Diatomaceous earth fact sheet.*
http://npic.orst.edu/factsheets/degen.html#whatis

NSW Government (n.d.). *What is Equine Influenza?*
https://www.dpi.nsw.gov.au/animals-and-livestock/horses/health-and-disease/influenza/what-is-equine-influenza

Oakland Veterinary (2019, September 27). *Retrospective: A Brief History of Veterinary Medicine.* https://www.ovrs.com/blog/history-of-veterinary-medicine/#:~:text=In%20the%201760s%2C%20Claude%20Bourgelat,animal%20medicine%20predating%209%2C000%20BC.

PennState Extension (2023, March 14). *Herb and Spice History.*
https://extension.psu.edu/herb-and-spice-history#:~:text=Herbal%20History&text=Herbs%20are%20mentioned%20in%20Genesis,Europe%20in%20the%20Middle%20Ages.

PennState Extention (2023, June 12). *How to take your horse's vitals.*
https://extension.psu.edu/how-to-take-your-horses-vital-signs

PennState Extention (2023, June 12). *Plants toxic to horses.*
https://extension.psu.edu/plants-toxic-to-horses

The Plaid Horse (2021, May 19). *Good Herbs and Vegetables for Your Horse.*
https://www.theplaidhorse.com/2021/05/19/good-herbs-and-vegetables-for-your-horse/#:~:text=Comfrey%20boosts%20the%20healing%20of,root%20of%20comfrey%20a%20day.

Pro Equine Grooms (n.d.). *Witch Hazel for Horses -Use with Caution.*
https://proequinegrooms.com/tips/health-and-well-being/witch-hazel-at-the-barn-use-with-caution/#:~:text=Generally%20speaking%2C%20you%20should%20not,witch%20hazel%20internally%20at%20all.

Quora (n.d.). *What Spices and Herbs are High in Zinc?*
https://www.quora.com/What-spices-and-herbs-are-high-in-zinc#:~:text=Some%20common%20spices%20and%20herbs,thyme%2C%20paprika%2C%20and%20fennel.

Rensberger, B. (1985, December, 27). *African chimps found to practice herbal medicine.* https://www.latimes.com/archives/la-xpm-1985-12-27-mn-25409-story.html

Reverdy (n.d.). *Turmeric.* https://www.reverdy.fr/en/turmeric-1kg

Rossdales Veterinary Surgeons (n.d.). *Wound Management.*
https://www.rossdales.com/services/sport-and-leisure-horses/routine-stable-visits/wound-management#:~:text=If%20the%20wound%20is%20large,how%20to%20apply%20a%20dressing.

Rose-Hip Vital (n.d.). *Dosage and Administration.*
https://rosehipvital.com/pages/equine-dosage

Royal Veterinary College (n.d.). *Equine Cushing's Disease.*
https://www.rvc.ac.uk/equine-vet/information-and-advice/fact-files/cushings-disease#panel-treatment-and-management

Ruff, S. (2016, July 7). *My Horse's Vet Bill is How Much?*
https://thehorse.com/18076/my-horses-vet-bill-is-how-much/

Rush, B. (2022, October). *Foul Pneumonia.*
https://www.merckvetmanual.com/horse-owners/lung-and-airway-disorders-of-horses/foal-pneumonia

Salatin, J. (n.d.). *'A Path Toward a Life Worth Living', The Homesteading Guide.*
pp. 173-177.

Schell, T. (n.d.). *Equine Stamina & Recovery; Influence of Two Key Herbs.* https://nouvelleresearch.com/index.php/articles/426-equine-stamina-recovery-influence-of-two-key-herbs

Scone Equine Hospital (n.d.). *Degenerative Joint Disease (DJD).* https://www.sconeequinehospital.com.au/blog/2021/08/10/degenerative-joint-disease/#:~:text=These%20signs%20may%20include%20joint,changes%20of%20osteoarthritis%20and%20lameness.

Scott Dunn's Equine Clinic (n.d.). *Mud Fever.* https://scott-dunns.co.uk/equine-advice/ailments-and-diseases/mud-fever/#:~:text=Mud%20fever%2C%20also%20known%20as,any%20leg%20can%20be%20affected.

SmartPak (n.d.). *Glossary of Active Ingredients.* https://www.smartpakequine.com/learn-health/horse-supplement-ingredients

Spaulding, C.E. (2010). *Veterinary Guide for Animal Owners.* pp. 182-183

Spaulding, C.E. (2010). *Veterinary Guide for Animal Owners.* pp. 191

Spaulding, C.E. (2010). *Veterinary Guide for Animal Owners.* pp. 200-203

Spaulding, C.E. (2010). *Veterinary Guide for Animal Owners.* pp. 204-206

Spaulding, C.E. (2010). *Veterinary Guide for Animal Owners.* pp. 207-208

Spaulding, C.E. (2010). *Veterinary Guide for Animal Owners.* pp. 209-210

Spaulding, C.E. (2010). *Veterinary Guide for Animal Owners.* pp. 211

Spaulding, C.E. (2010). *Veterinary Guide for Animal Owners.* pp. 212-115

Spaulding, C.E. (2010). *Veterinary Guide for Animal Owners.* pp. 216

Spaulding, C.E. (2010). *Veterinary Guide for Animal Owners.* pp. 217

Spaulding, C.E. (2010). *Veterinary Guide for Animal Owners.* pp. 218

Spaulding, C.E. (2010). *Veterinary Guide for Animal Owners.* pp. 219-220

Spaulding, C.E. (2010). *Veterinary Guide for Animal Owners.* pp. 221

Spaulding, C.E. (2010). *Veterinary Guide for Animal Owners.* pp. 222-223

Spaulding, C.E. (2010). *Veterinary Guide for Animal Owners.* pp. 224-225

Spaulding, C.E. (2010). *Veterinary Guide for Animal Owners.* pp. 226-227

Stronach, E. (2023, October 26). *Kelp for Horses: Uses and How to Feed.* https://madbarn.com/kelp-for-horses/

Stronach, E. (2023, December 15). *6 Research-Backed Benefits of Turmeric for Horses [Review].* https://madbarn.com/turmeric-benefits-for-horses/#:~:text=A%20dose%20of%20up%20to,without%20adverse%20effects.

Suttleworth, B. (2012, December 21). *Feeding Your Horse Ginseng.* https://www.horseandpethealth.com/feeding-your-horse-ginseng/#:~:text=The%20dose%20depends%20on%20the,grams%20should%20be%20taken%20daily.

Team Acko (2023, December 11). *Overview of Zinc and Ayurvedic medicine.* https://www.acko.com/health-insurance/zinc-ayurvedic-medicine/

Texas Horseman (2023, November 15). *Equine Encephalomyelitis: Understanding the "Sleeping Sickness".* https://www.thetexashorseman.com/2023/11/15/equine-encephalomyelitis-understanding-the-sleeping-sickness/

Tizzard, I. (2022, October). *The Immune System of Horses.* https://www.merckvetmanual.com/horse-owners/immune-disorders-of-horses/the-immune-system-of-horses#:~:text=The%20immune%20system%20consists%20of,immune%20system%20includes%20several%20organs

University of Minnesota Extension (n.d.). *Back Pain in Your Horse.* https://extension.umn.edu/horse-health/back-pain-your-horse#:~:text=Talk%20to%20your%20chiropractor%20about,area%20and%20relieve%20muscle%20spasms.

University of Minnesota Extension (n.d.). *Salmonella in Horses.* https://extension.umn.edu/horse-health/salmonella-horses#:~:text=Salmonella%20can%20upset%20the%20gut,if%20your%20horse%20is%20infected.

USDA (2023, June 30). *Equine Infectious Anemia (EIA).* https://www.aphis.usda.gov/aphis/ourfocus/animalhealth/animal-disease-information/equine/eia/equine-infectious-anemia#:~:text=Equine%20Infectious%20Anemia%20(EIA)%20is,acute%20phase%20of%20the%20infection.

USDA (2022, December 4). *West Nile Virus (WNV).* https://www.aphis.usda.gov/aphis/ourfocus/animalhealth/animal-disease-information/equine/wnv/west-nile-virus

U.S. Food and Drug Administration (2023, June 12). *FDA announces transition of over-the-counter medically important antimicrobials for animals to prescription status.* https://fda.gov/animal-veterinary/cvm-updates/fda-announces-transition-over-counter-medically-important-antimicrobials-animals-prescription-status

USP (2023). *U Publication Herbs SP.* https://www.usp.org/search?search_api_fulltext=publication%20herbs

Vedantu (2023, December 22). The male gender of 'mare' is 'horse'. https://www.vedantu.com/question-answer/the-male-gender-of-mare-is-horse-class-11-biology-cbse-60a6518ed4d0c6770f0dad53

Verm Oust (2019). *Equine-Horse wormer instructions.* https://vermoust.com/equine-horse-wormer-instructions/

Wishgarden (2018, July 9). *Herbs Natural Remedies for Insect Bites and Stings.* https://www.wishgardenherbs.com/blogs/wishgarden/natural-remedies-insect-bites-stings

Woo, C. (2012). *Herbal Medicine.* https://www.sciencedirect.com/topics/agricultural-and-biological-sciences/herbal-medicines

WorldHorseWelfare (n.d.). *Mites: How to Treat Them in Horses.* https://www.worldhorsewelfare.org/advice/mites-how-to-treat-them-in-horses

Wormers-Direct (2023, August 29). *Beneficial Herbs for Horses.* https://wormers-direct.co.uk/blog/beneficial-herbs-for-horses/

The Yale Ledger (2022, March 28). *What are the Benefits of Herbal Medicine?* https://campuspress.yale.edu/ledger/what-are-the-benefits-of-herbal-medicine/#:~:text=In%20contrast%2C%20herbal%20medicines%20are,avoid%20their%20possible%20side%20effects.

Young, A. (2020, March 23). *Laminitis.* https://ceh.vetmed.ucdavis.edu/health-topics/laminitis#:~:text=Laminitis%20is%20damage%20and%20inflammation,the%20other%2C%20connecting%20the%20two.

Young, A. (2021, March 29). *Tetanus.* https://ceh.vetmed.ucdavis.edu/health-topics/tetanus#:~:text=An%20inability%20to%20open%20the,become%20very%20sensitive%20to%20touch.

Young, A. (2020, August 10). *Strangles.* https://ceh.vetmed.ucdavis.edu/health-topics/strangles#:~:text=Strangles%20is%20a%20highly%20contagious,clinical%20signs%20than%20older%20horses.

Young, A. (2020, August 28). *Eastern Equine Encephalitis (EEE).* https://ceh.vetmed.ucdavis.edu/health-topics/eastern-equine-encephalitis-eee

Young, A. (2020, August 28). *Salmonellosis.* https://ceh.vetmed.ucdavis.edu/health-topics/salmonellosis#:~:text=The%20clinical%20signs%20of%20Salmonellosis%20in%20adult%20horses%20can%20include,transmitting%20it%20to%20other%20horses.

www.ingramcontent.com/pod-product-compliance
Lightning Source LLC
Chambersburg PA
CBHW062313290526
45794CB00005B/1784